Marshaling Support to Survive Breast Cancer

Self-talk, Girl-talk, Doctor-talk
A Memoir (2008)

Cheron Joy Mayhall

Outskirts Press, Inc.
Denver, Colorado

Outskirts Press, Inc.
http://www.outskirtspress.com

ISBN: 978-1-4327-3660-6

Outskirts Press and the "OP" logo are trademarks belonging to Outskirts Press, Inc.

PRINTED IN THE UNITED STATES OF AMERICA

DEDICATION

For Bill, my husband and best friend

In memory of Lucy, for her extraordinary
canine comfort

ACKNOWLEDGEMENTS

My heartfelt gratitude to all the people who supported my return to wellness. They formed a protective cocoon around me while I healed and learned to thrive again. Special thanks for the encouragement and critique of friends and colleagues in my writers group: Dusty, Evelyn, Mary and Willean. Also to Frances, who provided her special insights as a writer, counselor and breast cancer patient. These people make up the cast of characters you will meet reading my memoir.

For Karen —
With gratitude for
our long-time friendship
(remember Disneyland in 1960!?).
Love —
Cheryn
12/31/08

PREFACE

It didn't matter that I knew cancer to be an equal-opportunity disease. I'd seen good, health-conscious, God-loving folks suffer with cancer just as often as people who abused their bodies or were mean-spirited. Even little children with no apparent family history could die of cancer. Still, I didn't plan on the "Big C" getting me. I'd just turned 61 and thought my diet and exercise habits were very good, for an aging matron! My preventative regimen for health care had been excellent. I'd had all my shots. On the rare occasion I became ill, I treated the symptoms to regain health. As my body parts wore out, I went in for repairs.

Just the same, cancer found a hospitable spot in my body. In my left breast, to be specific. Alas, I wasn't to be among the seven lucky women to be spared in our society where one woman in eight will have breast cancer in her lifetime. The challenge for each afflicted person is to figure out the course of treatment best suited to confronting and conquering this great scourge of modern times. Cancer is very frightening, yet I knew the statistics for breast cancer cure to be positive and promising.

When an unexpected crisis like cancer slaps you across the face, it's necessary to wake up and take notice of the support within and around you – to confront your disease aggressively. As a teenager I had memorized a Bible verse that became my mantra from then on: "God did not give us a spirit of timidity but a spirit of power and love and self-control." II Timothy 1:7. In times of trial, I am inspired to marshal my support and act boldly – to take the bull by the horns.

First, I had to wrap my mind and spirit around the reality of my disease, and then muster all the internal and external support available to accompany me on the long path to wellness. I needed to "get my attitude right." I would have to plumb the depths of my life experience and believe this challenge could be overcome, just as other obstacles had been. I engaged in constant conversations with myself – "self-talk" – to rise above fear and despair. Importantly, my self-talk comes from my spiritual essence, which includes prayer and an absolute conviction that God gives me strength and power through trials and tribulation.

Help also came from garnering the support of friends, relatives and other acquaintances. In the arena of breast cancer, there is clearly a well-established sisterhood. At the time of my diagnosis, I knew several women who had survived breast cancer and only three who had died of it. I wasted no time getting myself adopted into the family of survivors. The information and encouragement they provided was invaluable. But I didn't stop with this cancer-knowing circle of friends. I shared my journey with just about anyone who I thought would listen and respond with compassion. A counselor-educator by profession, I am comfortable with self-disclosure as a therapeutic and teaching tool. One efficient way I shared my inner thoughts, or self-talk, was through periodic health updates I emailed to friends and relatives. I assumed they'd be interested in what I was thinking and doing in response to my cancer.

Most of my in-depth conversations were "girl-talk" with women of all ages. I drew great strength from those who had shared my experience. Of course, men can get breast cancer, too, although I never met one who had. It is overwhelmingly a female disease. However, there were men who also fit this category of friend and confidant. They shared the same depth of concern and caring as the "girls." My husband – my best friend – is my greatest support and sounding board. I have other supportive male friends as well. Among them are several pastors, co-workers, and husbands of breast cancer survivors. Thankfully, talking about one's breast health is no longer re-stricted by Victorian standards of modesty. Caring men can be engaged in helpful conversation about breast cancer with no fear that they hold a pornographic view of breasts, which is so prevalent in the media.

The third category essential to healing is the cadre of health professionals. I consider "doctor-talk" of equal im-portance to self-talk and girl-talk/friend-talk. Thousands upon thousands of medical and para-medical practitioners have now developed high levels of expertise in the field of oncology. Cancer patients may avail themselves of the benefits from a vast and ever-expanding body of clinical research. The patient can become an educated partner in pursuing positive outcomes from treatment. I started by carefully questioning trusted acquaintances to gather names of doctors and programs they trusted with their cancer care. In this way, I found providers who encouraged me to par-ticipate actively in the management of my disease. There were critical decisions to be made without delay. I needed advisers with whom I could trust my life.

Having a supportive spouse or significant other cannot be overrated. My doctor-husband, Bill, figures prominently in all three realms of support. Since he's been my number-one fan for two-thirds of my life, my inner voice or self-talk is much affected by our shared history. He's been the best kind of friend, never pandering to my self-pity or weakness, but encouraging and enabling me to be strong and confident. If I truly need him beside me, he's there. If I can handle my own problems reasonably well, he lets me be independent and appreciates my accomplishments. He takes a no-nonsense, scientific approach to health and keeps current with the medical literature.

This book chronicles a critical period in my life, begin-ning with diagnosis and ending ten months later when I was able to articulate the belief that I'd beaten breast cancer. I found and used resources I hadn't realized were available –

until that day when the tumor changed my life forever. Hopefully this book will provide some information and inspiration to empower others facing cancer, either personally or on behalf of loved ones.

ABOUT THE AUTHOR

Dr. Mayhall retired in 1997 after a 30-year career as a professional counselor, specializing in support for families raising children with disabilities and health impairments, and families grieving the death of a child. After graduation from Pacific University in Oregon, she worked as a Peace Corps Volunteer in Honduras to improve the lives of toddlers and their impoverished families in a mountain village.

Cheron was a medical social worker for teaching hospitals in Texas and New Mexico, and then worked with school children on the Navajo reservation before settling in Oregon to raise her family. In 1982, she graduated from Oregon State University with a Ph.D. in Counseling and Adult Education. In 1983-84, she founded the Coalition in Oregon for Parent Education (COPE) where she served for thirteen years as Executive Director. She served on the governing bodies of numerous state, regional and national organizations and agencies, including the National Parent Network on Disability. She was President of the American Society for Deaf Children from 1999 to 2002, and was awarded ASDC's most prestigious honor, the Lee Katz Award, in 2005.

Cheron lives with her husband and pets in Port Townsend, WA. They have three adult children and one grandson. In 2006 she published her first memoir, "The Bridge Is Love: A Journey Through Grief to Joy After the Death of a Child" (Trafford.com/05-1239). Besides writing, reading and volunteer work, her interests include travel and biking. In retirement she has been President of her county's Habitat for Humanity affiliate. Among other volunteer endeavors, she continues working in support of church missions at home and abroad.

SELF-TALK, GIRL-TALK, DOCTOR-TALK

Ready or not, life happens

Okay, stay calm; be conversant and try to sound intelligent.[1]

"So, is it a good idea to have the mass removed surgically even if it's benign?" I asked the young man sticking the needle into my left breast. Always the optimist, I wasn't ready to use the word "malignant" until the test results were unequivocal.

"Oh, you're going to want this removed for sure," replied the doctor as he carefully studied the monitor.

Oh, no! That isn't the reply nor the tone of voice I'd hoped to hear! I think I won't ask any more questions right now.

This was the third in a series of focused breast exams since Halloween day, 2003. It started with my annual, routine mammogram and escalated to a guided ultrasound on November 17, and the needle biopsy November 25. During my routine, annual physical exam in July, my primary doctor found nothing unusual during his manual, clinical examination of my breasts. I had followed up with breast self-exams (BSE) on August 1, September 1, and October

---

[1] Italicized passages denote my "self-talk" or inner voice. This includes thoughts shared through correspondence with friends and relatives, and my prayers.

1, discovering nothing remarkable.

Now, lying there and hearing this radiologist's straight-forward reply, a twinge of fear broke through my protective shield of optimism and confidence. I guess I'd expected his words to be more encouraging – "Don't worry. You'll be fine. " – but my brain knew I'd come to this cancer specialty clinic for the whole truth, and nothing but the truth.

I need to talk to Bill. He's my rock when my own solid base is eroding or shattering. I need his help to lift me out of this quicksand of doubt and fear.

Ginger greeted me in the waiting room with smiling words but questioning eyes. She had agreed on short notice to be my driver for this procedure in a facility 45 miles away from our small town. One of her close friends had come along, and the three of us had preceded the appointment with a frivolous shopping trip to the mall in Silverdale. A fun-filled outing with the girls then, incidentally, a little diagnostic procedure to rule out disease and confirm good health. Ginger told me of her experience when the doctor examined suspicious lumps in her breasts as they hung down like pendulums through a metal opening in the exam table. We'd laughed about that image.

"I'm feeling fine," I told the girls, "but they didn't make my boobs hang through a hole! No pain; I'm just a little woozy, and I have a bulky dressing to decrease swelling and bruising." I pushed back my shoulders and exaggerated my bust line for comic relief.

Let's just get home. I need to talk with Bill. And I need to start thawing the turkey, making the stuffing, setting the table, making the pies...Thanksgiving is day after tomorrow.

On the drive home to Port Townsend, I told my friends

what the doctor had said, then added, "But I'm pretty sure it's just a cyst and a little surgery will solve the problem. The lab results won't be ready until Friday and I have to prepare a feast for dinner guests both Thursday and Friday. I'll call you, Ginger, when I know more. Thanks for being my chauffeur."

My schedule of volunteer work and holiday preparations was already full without these added medical demands. Sensing the approach of an overwhelming tidal wave of confusion, I assumed the role of dutiful patient, letting my physician-husband carry some of the burden involving medical inquiries. He is tenacious about helping people toward wellness. I needed to be his primary patient now.

Bill gets impatient with unnecessary delays in treatment. Whereas my demeanor tends to be calm and never hysterical, Bill was already agitated because my diagnostic process was too slow. I'd had the routine mammogram on October 31. Two weeks transpired before I was informed by phone about the suspicious spot on my left breast x-ray. I took the first available appointment for the local radiologist to perform a guided ultrasound on November 17. Having heard no report of those findings, I realized a festering anxiety in my body, so I called my own doctor on November 24. He referred me for the needle biopsy. Ironically, it was in the afternoon mail of November 28 that I received written notice regarding my Halloween mammogram at our local hospital, "...change in breast appearance needs further study..." By then I already had a diagnosis of cancer and was scheduled for surgery.

"Dr. Stowe suggests I call Silverdale to make an appointment for biopsy after the Thanksgiving holiday," I reported to Bill that Monday afternoon, November 24.

"Give me the number," Bill commanded. He immediately phoned the secretary, securing an appointment for me the next day. "You'll need to stop taking your low-dose aspirin to reduce bleeding and bruising. They'll call you later today with more pre-op instructions." His hug assured me we'd be a dynamic duo in confronting this new assault, as had been the case during our 36 years of challenges as a couple and family.

That's taken care of. But, first, I have an appointment this afternoon to discuss a critique of the first chapter of my memoir. Then a meeting at Ginger's with the young family we're co-sponsoring for a Habitat house. I'll be home by four so I can contact the biopsy people if I've missed their call. Save Tuesday for Silverdale... Laura arrives home from Oregon Tuesday night. We'll have Wednesday to prep for turkey day after working my morning shift at the Habitat re-sale store. Keeping busy and distracted always helps me muscle through fear and worry. What's that quote? "Worry is like sand in an oyster: a little makes a pearl – too much will kill the animal."

My pre-op instructions included locating a driver since the anesthetic might impair my ability. Bill said, apologetically, "I'm sorry, Cheron. I have to work Tuesday in Oregon so I can't take you."

"That's okay," I assured him, "I'll ask Ginger or Mary to drive me. I'm sure one of them will be available. Don't worry. I'll be fine."

He knows I like to feel independent and in control. He trusts my competence, even when I'm a bit rattled. Besides, he knows my faith is strong and I trust God's guidance. He tells me how he brags about his "low-maintenance wife." I can handle this part without him...with a little help from my friends.

Ginger had replied with her characteristic, "Sure, I'm happy to help." She could always be depended upon to perceive the true needs of her friends, and willing to change her plans to be accommodating. "We can use a Silverdale trip to shop for last-minute Thanksgiving groceries, and maybe shop some Christmas sales at the mall." Her company made me almost look forward to the outing. Besides, I had a list of items I needed to buy for our younger daughter's graduation party on December 13. Tuesday wasn't going to be a one-hundred-percent serious or gloomy day. And, in fact, it wasn't. The test was completed and the results were pending.

Bill and our other daughter, Laura, arrived home from Oregon late Tuesday to inspirit me after a too-long afternoon and evening alone with my thoughts.

Why do the lyrics of "Hey, Look me Over"[2] keep singing through my brain? I haven't sung that song in decades – not since the sixties when it was the performance opener for our college quintet. I can just see the five of us in our flowered jackets, smiling broadly with hand and body motions to enhance the song's message: Becky and I at first soprano, Dorothy and Sue singing second, and SallyJo giving depth with alto. Hmmm...how about that?! I do believe my memories are trying to tell me something: When feeling down, be assertive and optimistic. Take charge of your behavior and emotions.

Laura, age 25, came to spend the long holiday weekend

2

"Hey, look me over; lend me an ear. Fresh out of clover, mortgaged up to here. But don't pass the plate, folks, don't pass the cup. I figure whenever you're down and out the only way is up. And I'll be up like a rosebud, high on the vine. Don't thumb your nose, bud, take a tip from mine. I'm a little bit short of the elbowroom, but let me get me some. And look out world here I come!" (from the Broadway musical, "Wildcats") with us. I hadn't told our children anything about my medical situation, choosing not to concern them with uncertainties. Laura and I joined Ginger and other volunteers to staff the Habitat re-sale store on Wednesday morning, then the two of us spent the afternoon measuring, chopping and baking in preparation for Thanksgiving dinner.

I'd related to Bill my instructions to call Dr. Stowe on Friday morning for results of the biopsy. That's the protocol: labs and specialists prefer to channel their findings back through the patient's primary physician. If there's bad news to share, or results that spark many questions, it's expected that one's own doctor is in a better position to provide the follow up. So, we determined to put it out of our minds as best we could until Friday – to enjoy the holidays with our daughters and their guests.

Katie, our youngest at 24, arrived Thursday morning with her brindle greyhound, Lexi. I was just finishing setting the table for six. Two of her friends from Americorps and the Coast Guard arrived by noon, delighted by the delicious aroma of roasting turkey, expressing their gratitude for the invitation to share our feast and family tradition.

The inevitable stress of waiting for medically significant news was eased by the warmth and humor of entertaining a houseful of young people in a holiday spirit. Counting our blessings overshadowed my fears and misgivings. We ate too much, watched football on TV, and played Scrabble. We were genuinely tired at bedtime. But sleep was elusive with the diagnosis just hours away.

I called Dr. Stowe's office at 8:30 a.m. Friday, only to hear a recorded message informing me that the office was closed for the holiday weekend. I went through the hospital switchboard to contact the doctor covering his practice. He said he couldn't access phone or fax messages locked in Dr. Stowe's office.

Okay. Now I'm getting stressed out. How can I be as-

sertive and knowledgeable about my health care if I can't get these answers? Ugh! I hate feeling like a powerless victim. What to do... More lyrics from "Hey, Look Me Over" invading my thoughts: "Nobody in the world is ever without a care; how can you win the world if nobody knows you're there?" That's it – we're calling the Silverdale lab right now!

"This is Dr. Mayhall," Bill said with authority. "Let me speak with the radiologist in the lab." Moments later he was discussing my biopsy results with the doctor, who just happened to be viewing my tissue specimens under the microscope.

Bill looked at me across his desk. "It's cancer. The tumor is still small, less than two centimeters, but it needs to be removed. I'll call Salem to see how soon they can get you on the surgery schedule. Is that okay?"

"Of course," I said, grateful that he had a plan of action while I was momentarily stunned and struggling to think straight. I wandered down the hall to where Laura was watching the big holiday parade televised from downtown Seattle. I waved to catch her eye because she is deaf.

Squarely confronting my demons has always worked best for me. No easy way to share bad news like this. I don't know the sign language vocabulary to discuss cancer. I'll have to fingerspell. Laura's smart; she'll get it. And not fatalistic, so she'll handle it okay.

"I have breast cancer," I signed and spelled, pointing to the area on my breast in which the tumor was discovered. She asked me how I knew. I related to her some details of the testing and the diagnosis received only moments earlier. "Your dad is making an appointment for an operation to get the growth removed. We'll get it taken care of." She nodded and returned to watching TV.

7

Aware that Katie was at the computer in the next room, and knowing she had overheard the investigative phone conversations I'd been having, I moved on to discuss the situation with her. She stood up, gathering me in a comforting embrace. "Oh, Mom, are you feeling okay?"

A hug...I needed that! Depend on Katie to sense my fear. I need to reassure her.

"Well, I don't feel sick, only scared; maybe sad, and a little angry. I'm sorry this has come up now, with the holidays ahead of us, and your graduation in two weeks. Bummer, huh?"

"Will surgery cure the cancer?" she asked as her eyes filled with tears.

"That'll start the process, but the treatment will probably be more extensive. Some women have just the lump removed; some have the whole breast removed, or maybe both breasts. There are oral medicines and chemical treatments like blood transfusions. My friend, Dorle, goes to Seattle for chemo infusions every few weeks. I think she also had radiation treatments. At any rate, I'm not canceling any of our plans as long as I'm feeling okay. Dad and I will make some calls to get more information. I'll let you know what we find out."

I'll get by with a little help from my friends

I need to call Sara. She was in treatment all last year and now she looks fabulous – healthier than ever. I'll have to call her office. Hopefully she hasn't left town for the holiday weekend. I need to talk with someone who's been through this.

I'd been acquainted with Sara for several years through our joint activities with the Habitat for Humanity affiliate, and because she and her husband, Ed, were our insurance agents. We currently served together on Habitat's Family Partnership committee, which Sara co-chaired. In September she had sent around an email inviting others and me to Tuesday potluck lunches at the home of Dorle Campbell. Dorle, who was a retired schoolteacher and very active in Habitat, now had metastatic cancer and a poor prognosis after breast cancer cells had spread to her liver.

Typical of Dorle's indomitable spirit, she had decided to surround herself with friends, fellowship and wholesome food, encouraging all comers to gather in her home every Tuesday at noon. It was called "Tuesdays with Dorle" on the model of *Tuesdays with Morrie* by Mitch Albom, a tender, true story of friendship, which was a popular book and a movie starring Jack Lemmon. I had gone to five or six of these warm and hope-filled luncheons. It was there that I had begun connecting with Sara on a deeper level. She had chosen to be very private through her journey with cancer treatment, and I had respected that choice. Until now.

I closed the door to my bedroom and cushioned my back with pillows as I dialed the number. "Sara, I'm glad to find you in town today. I'd like to talk with you about breast cancer. Can you spare a few minutes? Or, I could call you later, after work. I just got the diagnosis from my biopsy results."

"You have cancer," she said, confirming the reason for my call and opening our discussion. "Of course I can talk with you."

I brought her up to date on what had been happening and our initial plans for surgery. "We'll go to Salem, Oregon because Bill knows the medical community there. He had a private practice in orthopedic surgery in Salem for twenty-two years before I retired and we moved here to the Olympic Peninsula. My brother and my neighbor both died of pancreatic cancer within the past few years, but I haven't delved into any details regarding breast cancer."

Sara replied, "Well, I got through it and you will too. Right now I feel healthier and more hopeful than ever."

Sara does look terrific – slim, beautiful complexion and smile, pretty hair. Dorle looks good despite her ongoing treatment and bald head. Hmm...I wonder if I'm going to lose all my hair.

Sara gave me some details about her surgery, chemotherapy and radiation. I took notes to share with Bill. I learned about the study of axillary lymph nodes during surgery. In Sara's case, they had found cancer cells in her first lymph node. The surgeon dissected sixteen nodes through a separate incision. Each node was checked under the microscope until they felt sure they had removed any malignancy. Then the two incisions were sewn closed.

She told me she'd had two courses of chemo, each of which had different combinations of cancer-fighting drugs, and she'd undergone radiation. I asked her if it was better to have the whole breast removed. "That's a decision you'll have to make with your surgeon. Be sure Bill goes with you to all doctor appointments where you'll be making big decisions. You'll have to sort through a lot of information and make choices with significant consequences.

"Ed was beside me all the way. I felt I needed privacy and solitude to get through my cancer. He respected my wishes and protected me. I didn't feel comfortable being out in public where I might encounter a lot of questions, so we had regular out-of-town dates for a quiet dinner. It was nice, and we grew closer."

"Okay," I said, "I won't bother you further today. Thank you so much for sharing your story with me. I'm feeling better already."

"Don't ever hesitate to call," she said. "I'll be thinking of you and praying for you every day, anxious to hear how it's going. And, you're doing the right thing – calling other women who have experienced breast cancer. I wish I'd done more of that. I'll be watching for you at Dorle's house on Tuesdays, whenever you feel up to it. There are five or six breast cancer survivors in that group. They'll want to help. Take care, Cheron."

She's right. Even though we all know that Dorle's cancer is killing her, the women and men who gather there create a haven to nurture love and hope. I need to remain a part of that group. Dorle has chosen a good death, not allowing gloom and doom to defeat her spirit. She is so alive. So is Sara. I'm sticking with them!

Bill came into the bedroom to inform me that Dr. Strauss would operate at Salem Hospital on December 4. "You're scheduled to see him and get your pre-op work-up on Tuesday. I also got us an appointment to see an oncologist that day. Are you doing okay?"

"I just talked with Sara. She told me all about her surgery and other treatments. She went through it all just last year. Now she works full time, exercises everyday, and feels healthy and happy. I need to call Ginger and Mary to tell them what's up, then I'm going to call a couple of other survivors I know."

"Ask them for the names of local doctors they went to, in case you need chemo and radiation. Dr. Stowe probably has some oncologists in this area he refers patients to. You can ask him for suggestions on Monday."

"Thanks for getting me set up in Salem, honey," I said as I hugged him close. "I would have had a hard time figuring out what to do on my own, especially since it's a holiday weekend. Not having a plan would really be nerve-wracking."

"In my experience, one day's delay is one day too many when we're looking at cancer. Even if it's supposed to be slow growing, the anxiety it causes is harmful. If I discover cancer in one of my patients, I make an immediate referral to an oncologist. Sometimes to a surgeon as well. If that doctor can't get the patient in quickly, I refer elsewhere and I usually don't refer to that doctor again. Cancer can be a killer and people are very apprehensive. They need and deserve prompt care."

The doorbell rang at noon. Katie greeted her boyfriend, Ryan, who had come for lunch, as planned. His Coast Guard duties had kept him on the ship Thanksgiving Day, but he was looking forward to a feast of Thursday's leftovers. The two had been dating only a couple months so we didn't know Ryan very well. However, he was obviously a prince compared to some of the frogs Katie had dated in recent years. His sensitivity, respect and good manners were immediately apparent. His genuine smile made a person feel warm.

Before dinner I called Ginger and my neighbor, Mary. Both listened intently as I related the details of my diagnosis and our immediate plans for surgical intervention in Salem. They said they would be praying for me and offered to help in any way.

At the time we moved next door to Mary seven years earlier, my brother was struggling to survive pancreatic cancer. He had been dead only four years when Mary's husband, George, got the same diagnosis and died within weeks of his first symptoms. Part of our closeness was the grief we had shared. She was fifteen years my senior, but she was young at heart, witty, and generous in every way.

Ginger and I had met in an aerobics class at a local gym, also during the time my brother was dying. She noticed my sadness. Our ensuing conversation revealed that both of us had lost four-year-old sons in the 70's. Sharing that experience cemented a common bond upon which our close friendship was established. Ginger was my age. Our youngest children, a boy and a girl, were only a year apart.

We'd talked of matchmaking to get these offspring connected, but they were both away at college and both resistant to parental impositions regarding their friendships. We backed off.

Dianne was another close friend and neighbor, my age. As with Mary and George, she and her husband had built their retirement dream home on our street, but he lost his life to cancer not long afterward. Both women had faced their widowhood with courage and faith, inspiring others and nurturing an inclusive network of support in our community. I wanted to call Dianne now, but, since she knew nothing about my month of tests and wasn't waiting to hear from me, I decided it would have to wait.

Laura, Katie and Ryan have come to share the family holiday with Bill and me. Enough of this cancer business. It can wait while we re-run the Thanksgiving feast and enjoy some football "tube time." Come to think of it, I haven't eaten a bite since yesterday afternoon. We'd better get that refrigerator-full of food set out for consumption since we're likely to be in Oregon all next week.

Laura and I had made peanut butter pie as an alternative to pumpkin and mincemeat. This sweet treat capped a satisfying meal of turkey with all the trimmings, Round Two! Ryan's presence at the table helped keep the conversation upbeat and cancer-free. Katie told me later she'd shared the news of my diagnosis with him during a phone call earlier that morning. He'd offered to stay away, respectful of our family's need for time to digest the shocking news. "Oh, no," Katie told him, "Mom's looking forward to your visit. She needs you to come. I need you. Our whole family needs you!"

That day remains precious in my memory. Ryan was an integral part of the intense journey unfolding for our family. He supported Katie through her great sensitivity and sadness during the ensuing months. That supportive link also strengthened me. He encouraged Katie to spend weekends with me rather than stay behind with him. When they both had time off from their work as substitute teacher and Coast Guardsman, they'd come to cheer me. Sometimes they'd bring flowers or other small gifts; always they brought kindness and humor.

Too anxious to sleep more than a few hours, I was up early Saturday morning, checking my email – a comical electronic Thanksgiving greeting from Dianne and a notice about my forthcoming Trustees meeting at the church. I would call these folks after sun-up. It wasn't too early, though, to compose an email message to my three sisters in Seattle, Spokane and Florida.

Dear Alice, Mary and Connie: Well, Thanksgiving is behind us again. Our girls were here, plus a number of Katie's friends from Port Angeles. Two of her girlfriends from Bellingham also stopped by. So, we had turkey meals both Thursday and Friday. Now to forge ahead into December...

And the bad news is...yesterday I got confirmation of cancer in my left breast. I have had a number of tests since early November, and the results kept getting worse and worse. So, I am scared and sad and mad...a whole bunch of emotions keeping me awake at night. But, most of the time I try to stay rational and remember that I know many survivors. They are active and enjoying life, so that's my reason for hope.

We will leave for Oregon Monday for Tuesday appointments with the surgeon and oncologist, a number of pre-op lab tests, then the surgery on Thursday. We are hoping I can come home to heal by the end of next weekend. After that, it may be radiation and/or chemo, but we won't know until they've seen the extent of the cancer. We'll just have to go one day at a time and get through this. My doctor did not feel the lump during my annual exam in July, and I didn't find it on self-exam after that. It was the October 30 mammo that found something suspicious. Be sure you're checking this regularly, okay?

Well, sorry to share this negative news, but you would want to know, I'm sure. Keep me in your thoughts and prayers. Love, Cheron

I brewed the coffee and treated myself to a thin wedge of peanut butter pie just before eight o'clock. From my kitchen window I saw Dianne retrieve her newspaper from the curb. "Hello," said her distinctive, cheery voice on the phone line. Dianne had grieved with and for numerous loved ones during the six years we'd been acquainted, including her husband and her daughter's several miscarriages or stillbirths that ended those dreams of grandparenting. She remained strong and stable. I knew she'd want to know about my cancer.

"Good morning, Dianne. How was your Thanksgiving?" She related to me the good times with her married children and one infant grandson. I shared the highlights of two days with daughters and friends, then zeroed in on the news of my cancer.

"Oh, friend," she said, "I can't imagine what you're going through. How can I help? Do you need me to take care of the cat – or anything else – while you're in Oregon?" I thanked her for the offer but reminded her that our orange tabby, Thumb-purr, was self-reliant. If we left a good supply of food and water, he could come and go through the doggie door to get all his needs met.

"Okay, I'll watch for your return and I'll bring dinner. Does Mary know? She and I can cook for you if you don't feel up to it. I'll be praying you get good weather for the trip and for no complications from the surgery."

Buoyed by Dianne's heartfelt expressions of friendship and support, I called the chair of Trustees at the First Pres-

15

byterian Church to let him know I'd have to miss Wednesday's meeting. I thought I'd better relate the reason I'd need to be excused, which turned out to be a good decision. "Breast cancer, huh?" he said. "Here, let me have you talk to my wife. She's a survivor of many years." And, though I hardly knew the woman, Judy was soon sharing her success story and assuring me that life was, indeed, good after breast cancer.

Wow! Every single person I talk with improves my disposition – raises my hope. I feel like I'm on a roll (or is it a roller coaster?). If this keeps up I'll have so many prayers and good vibes coming my way, I can't help but have a good outcome from surgery. Thank you, God, for surrounding me with so many loving people.

Thumb-purr meowed for his breakfast just as Laura and Katie emerged from the downstairs bedrooms. Ryan and Bill joined us for coffee and bagels, after which I drove Ryan and Katie to the Habitat store in town. Ryan was hoping to find some secondhand house wares or furniture to outfit his new apartment in Port Angeles. I was glad to see Cameron staffing the cash register. She and I shared a seven-year history of volunteerism and board membership for Habitat and I knew she'd survived breast cancer. She'd attended a few of Dorle's potlucks.

"I was just diagnosed with breast cancer," I confided. No shoppers within earshot, she put her arm around my shoulders and proceeded to relate her experience. Now 66, she had been cancer-free for eleven years. Treatment choices had been far fewer a decade earlier, but her health had returned so she'd led a full and active life. She, like Sara, reminded me to involve Bill. "My husband shared in all the decision making. I never felt from him any of the rejection you'll read or hear about. My disease became <u>our</u> disease. My recovery has been as much his victory as my

16

own."

With Ryan and Katie headed back to Port Angeles, the house was quiet that afternoon – too quiet. Bill and Laura were enjoying down time, reading, napping, working on a laptop or watching TV in comfortable recliners. Full of nervous energy and unable to relax, I changed all the bed linen and started the laundry. Then I packed my suitcase for the week in Oregon. Thinking ahead to Katie's graduation party, I polished the silverware. Bill and I had been discussing getting a small dog to replace our old Dalmatian who'd died several weeks earlier. So, I surfed the Web in search of cocker spaniels needing adoptive homes. All this only partially succeeded in diverting my attention from the cancer.

I hate this nagging fear and anxiety. What did I do to deserve cancer? I'm feeling victimized. I, who have struggled all my life to avoid the victim mentality. Why me? Why not me? I had to grapple with the same questions when our son Scotty was killed, and when our other kids were identified as disabled or chronically ill. Same answer now as then: Life is not fair.

Yet, there's nothing to be gained by wallowing in self-pity or being immobilized by misfortune. "Get your attitude right!" Bill picked up that phrase mimicking an obnoxious televangelist in the 80s. We used it a lot when our teenagers would bellyache and complain. It usually turned crabbiness to laughter, conjuring up the image of the self-proclaimed faith healer strutting his stuff in front of an emotional, tent-revival audience.

Get my attitude right! What was it Nelson Mandela said about personal power? God's spirit is in every one of us. We were born to exercise that power so our light can shine and make the world a better place. No sniveling...no shirking your responsibilities. I don't suppose having cancer gives me a bye from that mandate. "We are powerful be-

17

yond measure" according to the great Mandela.

The words of South Africa's liberator had invaded my consciousness. His powerful 1994 inaugural message had inspired me before. He was speaking to me now.

I called my friend, Allie, with whom I shared a corner of the room where our neighborhood exercise class met three mornings a week. I recalled she'd had radical cancer surgery many years ago. It didn't seem to slow her down. She was older than I.

"So, what are you going to do about it, Toots?" was her reply when I shared my plight. She filled me in on details regarding her own cancer treatment, plus what she knew of other survivors. "It seems that every case is unique. What worked for me fifteen years ago won't be a good solution for you. So much progress has been made. What likely is the same for all of us is the experience of fear and helplessness. But you'll get through it just fine. Sounds like you've been diagnosed early and you have a plan to start treatment without delay. Do you feel like going to exercise class on Monday?"

"Sure," I replied. "I've got to keep my mind and body busy. Maybe I won't be able to exercise after the surgery, but I'm fine now. Well," I added, "my back and knees ache, as usual, but that hasn't stopped me yet."

"Okay, I'll see you Monday then. Call me if you come up with any more questions."

Sunday I arose early because I was scheduled to make presentations about our El Salvador mission project during both church services as well as for the adult Sunday school class. I'd traveled to Central America with two of the four teams sponsored by our church, working over several years with the impoverished families in a small village named Santa Elena. Bill and I had taken particular interest in helping Santa Elenans get a well drilled to supply clean water for drinking and hygiene. I'd learned Spanish in the Peace

Corps, which helped cross the language barrier, so I agreed to be the key person keeping tabs on the project via email and the Internet.

Normally I attended only late service, not the smaller, less formal early service. One of many differences in the order of worship was time allowed for Rev. Slater to move about the congregation with a microphone, asking worshippers to share their joys and concerns. I was surprised to find my hand raised to get his attention, never having been comfortable volunteering such information in this format. "I have just been diagnosed with breast cancer. Bill and I will leave tomorrow for Salem, OR, where I will have a pre-op work-up, then surgery next Thursday. Please keep us in your prayers." The pastor touched my shoulder with warm assurance. I heard a sigh from friends around me in the pews.

Well, that wasn't so hard. Feels good to get it out in the open. People here need to know I'll probably be distracted and less available until this gets sorted out. They'll put me on the prayer chain. I'll take all the support I can muster!

It was good to be able to share news about progress with the well-drilling project in El Salvador. It had been frustratingly slow to materialize, fraught with barriers involving funding, politics, weather, geology and geography of the region. Now it appeared there would soon be potable water flowing, and this had sparked additional activity wherein latrines and toilets were being installed, a new school was being built, electricity was coming into some residences, and roadway access to the village was greatly improved. For a while I could forget cancer and share the good news of Santa Elena. The church was forming a delegation to visit El Salvador the next summer. Unsure of whether or not I would be healthy enough to travel there, I nonetheless was willing and anxious to help with planning and to share my knowledge of the area and Spanish with those who would go. My three presentations came off well.

Bob, our pastor, was very helpful and compassionate, assuring me that the whole congregation would rally to support me through cancer treatment. After my presentation from the pulpit during the eleven o'clock service, I was about to leave the sanctuary when Bill and Judy Master beckoned to me. He was the chair of Trustees; she was his wife who'd survived breast cancer and coached me by phone the day before. They handed me an envelope, touched my hand and smiled empathetically. They'd faced and conquered breast cancer together. When I got to the car I opened the greeting card envelope and out fell a stone engraved with the word, "Courage." The Masters were sharing this tangible talisman, reminding me to stay strong. I would carry the stone in my pocket or purse through all the months of treatments ahead.

As I drove home from the church I searched my memories of how breast cancer had affected my life.

We've had our share of cancer in the family. Now that I think of it, in my lifetime many dear relatives have died: Grandma Gratia, Uncle Grant, my big brother, Alex, and maybe Aunt Hazel. None of these blood relatives had breast cancer, although no one seems to know for sure where grandma's cancer started. Cancer conversation seemed to be taboo for her generation, especially if it involved a woman's private parts. Thank God I'm not feeling such constraints. Oh, and my beloved Aunt Libby...she died of a breast cancer that ate through her chest while she refused treatment because of her Christian Science beliefs. That was about 1970, and I still grieve that she kept her illness a secret and that we weren't allowed to visit her in Montana. Libby was a summertime surrogate mother to me as a child and teen. She was one of the funniest and most joyful people I ever knew. She died in great pain, and I never got to say

20

good-bye.

I realized the tears were dripping off my chin as I drove into our garage. Taking a deep breath, I focused on Dorle and her cadre of friends so close by, many of whom were cancer survivors. The tightness in my chest and throat eased momentarily. Then I thought again of the wives of long-time friends, Darrell and Jim. These women had succumbed to their breast cancer, one three years earlier and the other about twelve. They were relatively young and beautiful women. I didn't see enough of them because they lived in California, but I could still get in touch with my sorrow for their husbands and children. It strengthened my resolve to face this new challenge aggressively, and with COURAGE. I fingered the stone lying in my lap. I perceived an infusion of power as I headed indoors. After a light lunch, I tried to watch a televised football game with Bill, but my body was exhausted. I napped peacefully in the recliner, unusual for me since I very rarely slept during daylight hours.

Before supper there was a knock at the front door. My neighbor, Allie, who'd had a mastectomy many years earlier, brought me a wrapped gift and a hug. Inside the package was a Precious Moments figurine of a chubby child standing with arms outstretched and boxing gloves on her fists. On her shirt was the pink ribbon symbol now widely associated with the campaign for breast cancer awareness and cure. The statuette was inscribed, "Life is Worth Fighting For." Allie remarked, "I don't know what possessed me to buy it a while back because I don't normally do things like that. But, here it is with my wishes that you'll get through this ordeal and come out stronger." I told her about the courage stone I'd received. She concurred with the advice to stay strong and "muscle" through the treatment. She was sure that I'd soon be able to call myself a cancer survivor. We smiled and hugged. She continued to chatter reassuring words as she disappeared down the block.

Before bed I thought of several more friends who I judged would want to know about my diagnosis, so I selected fifteen email addresses and dashed off a short note:

Hi: I'm writing this brief message to a select group of friends who I suspect would not want to be left out of the loop. After a month of testing, I was diagnosed on Friday with breast cancer. We will leave tomorrow morning for initial treatment in Oregon. Tuesday we have appointments with a surgeon and an oncologist, some pre-op tests, and then surgery on Thursday morning in Salem. Hopefully I'll be out of the hospital and home to recover before the end of the weekend.

I apologize for sharing this negative news as we enter this season of joy, but I need your encouragement and prayers. I'm working at staying optimistic. Of course, I'm a little sad and scared, but most of the time I can remind myself that I know, or know of, lots of women survivors. I have talked at length with four here in Port Townsend, each of whom had a different experience, but all have survived at least a year, and one more than fifteen years. I'll get back to you post-op. Love, Cheron, 11/30/03

Monday morning I headed for exercise class. It occurred to me that I was exercising matter over mind instead of the usual mind over matter. My thoughts and spirit were definitely droopy, but I was aware that my body felt no unusual pain in spite of the cancerous tumor in my breast. For six years I'd worked out regularly with this group of women, and more recently I'd added workouts at Curves on Tuesdays, Thursdays, and most Saturdays. I knew I needed physical exercise to curtail weight gain and maintain cardiopulmonary health, as well as to build flexibility and strength. Though my aging muscles and joints often ached,

I convinced myself that the situation would only worsen if I put on extra pounds and became more sedentary. Besides, these women had become a social support group. I missed them if I had to skip class for more than a few sessions.

Our capable and dedicated volunteer leader, Doris, put us through the paces for a full hour. I knew the routine well so my body kept going even when my mind wandered into the realms of cancer concern. We always closed every session with a group hug and sharing time, usually a joke or a review of the new movie or other activities going on in town. We kept up with the health and whereabouts of women who were absent, often sending greeting cards to cheer those who were struggling with some challenge. I felt totally at ease, perhaps even compelled, to share news of my current situation.

"Well, join the crowd," said one of the women. Four or five classmates identified themselves as breast cancer survivors. Three others spoke up about their diagnoses and treatments for a variety of other cancers. A sizeable proportion of the women in that circle had experiences, expertise and encouragement to share. Several of them told me anecdotes right there in the group, or later one-on-one. The sisterhood of survivors was growing exponentially all around me!

Dr. Stowe, my primary care doctor, called as soon as he read the biopsy report faxed to him from the lab in Silverdale. I brought him up to date on all that had transpired during the past few days, including our impending departure for surgery in Salem. "I know this is very emotional," he said. "But, we'll get you through it. What can I do to help right now?" I told him I'd need to drop by his office within the hour for copies of some reports in my medical file, which might alleviate the necessity for some of the pre-op testing. I asked him to be thinking of providers in the local area where I might be referred if I needed chemotherapy or radiation treatments. He and his nurse prepared a folder of relevant information I'd hand carry to Salem. They scheduled an appointment for me to see him a week after the surgery.

Cut it out!

During the five-hour drive to Salem, Bill and I had a chance to discuss what we were learning and thinking about this sudden new development in our lives. While I'd been gleaning information from women who had experienced breast cancer, he'd been talking by phone with doctors and reading the best literature he could find on the Internet site called "Medscape from WebMD." We realized that we had many important decisions confronting us within the next few hours and days. The most immediate question was, "lumpectomy" or "mastectomy?" Was it better to have the lump taken out, or to go ahead and remove the whole breast? We'd talked about this before in relation to other women, when it wasn't personal. We had concurred that removing the breast – even both breasts – was the way to go if it meant getting rid of the threat of all future breast cancer. Both of us still felt okay with that option.

"One of the women in my running group who has a family history of serious breast cancer finally decided to have both breasts removed," Bill remarked, "even before she had a diagnosis of malignancy. She'd dealt with some atypical findings and her doctors felt it was prudent to do the radical surgery. She got through it just fine. She's a good runner and apparently very healthy now."

He'd read that women choosing mastectomy usually didn't need chemo or radiation. That was a plus. We got a chuckle and much needed comic relief when he reported one study he'd read about a procedure to rebuild a woman's breasts using belly fat excised and folded up to the chest area. "Hey, you can have a tummy tuck and breast reconstruction at the same time!" I had always wished for a flatter tummy, and even more so in recent years as my skin began to sag and drag.

"One of the long-time survivors I've talked with didn't go through reconstructive surgery at all," I recounted. "She does just fine with a special bra and prosthesis. The only drawback she's told me about is discomfort undressing in public places, like the locker room at the swimming pool. Too many stares and questions have caused her to give up swimming, which she had always loved."

After settling into our motel in Salem, we met our friends, Noel and Myrna, for dinner at a restaurant. Both of them were pastoral counselors, but we knew them best as bicycle buddies with whom we'd shared adventures in the San Juan Islands and the Gulf Islands of British Columbia. I told them I was a little frightened but eager to consult with the surgeon and oncologist the next day so we could get the cancer out of my body. Noel apologized because he had a commitment out of town and wouldn't be able to visit me at the hospital in his role as chaplain. He assured me that another pastor would visit in his stead. I felt comforted just knowing they were pulling for me. I assured them I'd be fine.

Well, I WILL be fine! I'm basically pretty healthy. We've caught the tumor while it's still small. We're wasting no time getting to treatment. I've been hospitalized a dozen times before, if giving birth counts, although usually for elective rather than emergency procedures, which I guess cancer surgery is. I've never been afraid of hospitals or doctors. Hmm...there's definitely a tight feeling in my chest and stomach right now. Maybe that's fear, maybe not. Maybe it was the salad dressing or the clam chowder. Whatever. Tomorrow we'll get more answers. That'll be a relief, I think. God give me the power to forge ahead. Katie's graduation and party is less than two weeks from now.

I've got to be in shape to celebrate with her. In shape? That's funny. Good chance I'll be flat-chested by then, but I know I'll still feel that swelling in my breast for pride in her accomplishment. Guess we don't need breasts to feel a stirring in our souls!

Early Tuesday I dropped Bill off at his Salem office where he'd see his patients while I kept my hospital appointments for lab work, a chest x-ray and an EKG. These would help the surgeon and anesthesiologist ascertain whether or not my blood composition, lungs and heart were in shape to withstand the trauma of surgery. Every specialist who poked and prodded me through these routine procedures was sensitive and kind, yet I felt a shroud of sadness enveloping me.

Get your attitude right! You're a big girl and you've had all these tests before. One step at a time. When I get through this testing Bill and I will go together to see Dr. Strauss and the oncologist. We'll get some answers to plan next steps, and then I can relax for a day before the surgery. Right now I need to breathe deeply and walk tall. Lord God, I pray for your steady hand to guide me. Amen

I remembered a small poster a Native American friend once gave me when I faced some turmoil in my life. I knew the verse was meant to be calming and to inspire a peaceful spirit:

> Be still until the waters clear.
> Do nothing until the darkness ends.
> Rest until the storm clouds pass.
> Wait for winter's breath to die.
> Nature does not fight against itself...
> Nor does it dance when the music ends.

This is too funny: I remember telling people when I was small that I was related to Sitting Bull. I don't know where I got the idea, if someone else suggested it or it was a figment of my imagination. My parents grew up in Miles City, Montana, near the Little Big Horn Battle Ground. I'd been there a couple times. Maybe I'd romanticized my own connection to the warriors. Of course, I fancied myself an Indian maiden, a cross between Princess Summer-Fall-Winter-Spring on the Howdy Doody Show and Debra Paget's portrayal as Jimmy Stewart's love interest in "Broken Arrow." Right now it's doubtful I have the patience to make a good Indian!

Okay, I can calm myself in this moment, but I rebel at the idea of doing nothing to fight against this cancer. Please, God, you don't expect me to sit back and wait it out, do you? Aunt Libby waited faithfully while hoping her Christian Science beliefs would pull her through, but even with this deep faith the cancer killed her. I'm still angry that she died so young, without ever meeting my husband and children. I can't believe you would want me to accept this disease gracefully, without a fight. I still have a lot of things I want to do in this life. And I think they are things you would want me to do...mostly. Please help Bill and me to make the right decisions so I can be healthy and active again. Amen.

I realized I was engaging in behaviors common to the "bargaining" stage of grief work. I knew a lot about Dr. Elisabeth Kubler-Ross' theoretical stages through which terminal patients might pass while seeking a peaceful acceptance of their death. What I'd learned from my counseling practice was to guide clients through the stages of "denial" and "bargaining" so they could get quickly to the business of grieving, then on to peaceful resolution.

Hold on! Nobody has told me I'm going to die. Actually,

I don't believe it's come to that. Most women survive breast cancer, and I will too. It's not like me to dwell on the negative. I need to be realistic but hopeful about the surgery and treatment. It's not going to be fun, and it's going to put a monkey wrench in my plans for a while. Comedienne Gilda Radner called cancer "unfunny," and she was sure right about that. But, I'll get through it and be healthy again, like Allie, Judy, Cameron, Georgia and Sara. Time to get my butt over to Dr. Strauss' office to hear what he has to say.

Dr. Strauss turned out to be a cheery young fellow. After interviewing Bill and me, and discussing the results from the morning's tests, he recommended the conservative surgical approach of lumpectomy, i.e. removing just the cancerous tumor and a margin of tissue surrounding it. Bill and I still weren't willing to give up the consideration of total breast removal if that would improve the likelihood of cure. Dr. Strauss referred us to the oncologist to continue this discussion, but he was of the opinion that he could remove the malignancy and still conserve the breast at near its normal size and shape. He seemed enthusiastic for the opportunity to try.

The oncologist Bill had located was not so cheery, but I was glad he was available to counsel us on short notice. We learned from him that there was no evidence to show that mastectomy was preferable to lumpectomy with radiation. He gave us the facts but was unwilling to make the decision for us. He also took seriously his responsibility to impress upon cancer patients the gravity of the disease. He knew all the statistics about death and recurrence and metastasis. I guessed I'd not be so cheery, either, if it was my job, every single day, to level with patients and their families about the negative possibilities in facing cancer. He also educated us further about the need for lymph node exploration, and dissection if it was warranted. He knew the reputations of a clinical oncologist and a radiation oncologist in the Port

Townsend area, so we jotted a note about his recommendation in this.

"Sounds to me like surgery, radiation AND chemotherapy are the best bets to handle this lump in my breast," I summarized when we were back at the motel. "That's what Sara went through last year and what I've kind of been expecting to go through, too." I'd collected a big pile of literature about treatment options from every office or lab I'd visited that day. The hospital had also given me reading to do and forms to complete, so I had plenty of homework to keep busy until Thursday. Bill called Dr. Strauss to confirm our decision regarding the lumpectomy so he could plan his surgery schedule accordingly. Then I plunged into my reading in hopes of gaining a better understanding about the lymph node part of the operation.

Bill had a full schedule of patients to see on Wednesday, so I mapped out a plan to stay busy and active. I took my Curves guest pass to one of their franchises near our motel. The workout program and facilities are designed to build a woman's confidence and resolve to be the best she can be. There is beauty in the color and décor surrounding the stations of strength-building machines arranged in a circle. Music with a snappy beat keeps the muscles working and heart pumping during a thirty-minute workout that usually seems shorter, yet satisfying. I felt encouraged by the smiles of the staff and fellow exercisers. I read all the words of inspiration posted around the walls and taped to the windows. I left feeling stronger and more positive.

With the whole afternoon still ahead of me, I headed north on the highway for the outlet mall that was advertising dynamite pre-Christmas sales. I had some coupons that helped me determine which of the stores might have good buys. I window-shopped and circled in and through at least thirty stores before taking a couple small packages and my giant pretzel from the snack shop back to the car for the return to Salem.

I remember a feeling of being stalled that evening – like an airplane in a holding pattern, waiting for the journey to get underway. I wasn't sad or mad, just stuck, awaiting my fate. We'd done all we could to prepare. Now it was in someone else's hands. A whole team of doctors and other medical professionals awaited me the next morning, ready to help with this next step.

I'm ready, Lord. I believe you've led Bill and me to this place and this moment. Give me strength and courage for the 'morrow (waxing poetic!), and the patience and perseverance I'll need for months to come. Good night and Amen.

Bill checked me into the hospital before eight on Thursday morning. I was hungry and agitated for lack of my morning coffee, but otherwise feeling optimistic about the surgery that was to occur in a couple hours. After changing into my hospital duds I wrote in my journal and began reading a novel while awaiting visits from the doctors. A week earlier I had begun reading Ken Follett's *The Pillars of the Earth,* a welcome change from Solzhenitsyn's *Cancer Ward.* I found it ironic that I was attempting to plow through this depressing cancer story at the time I got my diagnosis. Having very intentionally curtailed my volunteer activities to try my hand as a writer, beginning in September, I had also pledged myself to reading more of the acclaimed works of literature and familiarizing myself with the best contemporary authors. I'd never read this Russian writer's award-winning book about the "gulag," but I'd found *Cancer Ward* at the Habitat second-hand bookstore and decided it would serve my purposes. In light of this new diagnosis, I wasn't foolish enough to test my perseverance and optimism by proceeding to spend my free time reading a novel about cancer patients in a sanitarium with little hope of survival. Reading *Pillars* was a joy by comparison.

It turned out to be a very long waiting period during which my optimism wavered and almost died. A tech came to insert an IV, the nurse checked my vital signs a couple times, and various other personnel dropped by to discuss anesthesia and a procedure I'd heretofore not been apprised of – insertion of a wire in the tumor. I was told this would help the surgeon locate the malignancy with greater precision. By the time our former pastor came by as Noel's substitute chaplain, I had to admit I was feeling depressed and teary. He acknowledged the appropriateness of those emotions. We prayed together for God's calming presence and His guidance for the hospital professionals who would provide this first approach to treatment.

From my curtained cubicle in the prep area I had a view of the bathroom. I recognized a familiar face going in and out, so called to see if it was a former colleague from my days working in Oregon special education programs. Hilda and I had served on a couple boards or committees together, and we both advocated for disability rights at the Oregon Legislature. Our daughters went to the same schools. Now she told me that she was about to undergo surgery for a brain tumor, but she'd had the same procedure before and was optimistic about the outcome. She appeared confident and fearless.

Well, that certainly helps to put things in perspective. I've just got this little lump in my breast while she has a recurrent growth on her brain. I need to practice what I've preached to my children: If you think you've got it bad, just look around and you'll always find a person whose facing a greater challenge with fewer resources. It's no coincidence that Hilda just happens to be in the surgery queue with me today. Thank you, God, for sending this reminder. And be with Hilda and her family today.

Between 12:30 and 1:30 the wire-insertion was accomplished and I had a follow-up mammogram to be sure it provided the guidance Dr. Strauss would need to excise the tumor. Surgery started shortly thereafter and I didn't feel a thing until the anesthetic started to wear off at 4 p.m.

As I awoke, I felt hot tears rolling down both cheeks into my ears while the recovery room nurse caressed my hand. I was experiencing the worst migraine headache in history with excruciating pain when I tried to open my eyes. "What's wrong?" she asked. "Are you having physical pain, or is it the other?" I was in too much distress to go beyond, "My head's going to explode!" They tried a variety of painkillers with little success before moving me to my hospital room. Being wheeled down the halls and lifted from gurney to bed was agonizing. I realized later that "…is it the other?" was probably the nurse's attempt to acknowledge my rational fear of cancer and having part of my breast removed. Neither of these concerns could hold a candle to the monster headache that completely debilitated me for twenty-four hours in the aftermath of surgery.

The pain at the surgical sites of the tumor excision and lymph node exploration was inconsequential compared to migraine symptoms of vertigo, vomiting and heavy sweats. Bill came to spend the evening with me but couldn't stand watching my misery. The nursing staff could call him at the motel when I became less dependent on sedation and more coherent. During the long night I began to sense hunger and thirst but was unable to hold anything down. Bill and Dr. Strauss could plainly see I wasn't ready for discharge anytime Friday. It took another twenty-four hours for me to stabilize enough to be taught the routine of self-care I'd be following at home. One of my former co-workers and our Salem neighbors, all close friends, came by my hospital room with good wishes, helping to pass the time and get me up and moving.

There was a long drainage tube coming out of a hole under my arm. It led to a sack pinned to my gown below my waist. The sack had a suction mechanism designed to remove excess lymph build-up in my traumatized arm and breast tissues. I would have to clear the tube and empty the sack of any fluid at least twice a day. The day I left the hospital the drainage measured 155ccs, and the target was to be below 10ccs before the drain could be removed. Eleven days later it was reduced to 24ccs, but then I went back for a second operation and it shot up to 51ccs post-op. It was a "yucky nuisance," I told friends who inquired, but it caused no pain. In fact, after Christmas I was able to do most of the routines in my exercise class with little problem, despite the tube and sack apparatus beneath my workout clothes.

The importance of using my left arm was impressed upon me. I routinely did the prescribed exercises with an elastic band attached to the top of my closet door, to keep the range of motion in my shoulder and build strength in my left arm – my dominant side. I was starting to feel pretty good by December 7, at which time I learned that the margin around the tumor excision site was deemed "insufficient" as viewed under the microscope. I needed a second surgery to carve out a little more tissue. This operation could be done on an outpatient basis in Salem by the same surgeon. It was scheduled for December 18.

On December 8, I felt well enough to do a couple loads of laundry, after which I wrote an email update to the group of friends who I'd informed about the surgery:

Hi all: We have two doctor friends, both named Richard, who have told me, in so many words, that I'm a "tough old bird." Okay, I suppose it's true that I'm no longer a tender young chick, but I'll happily ascribe to any characteristics that help me beat this cancer. I expect to survive long enough to see at least one grandchild graduate from high school, and that means I'll have to stick around until I'm 80 (hopefully even longer).

Here's the good news: It appears the cancer did not infiltrate my lymph system. Twenty-one lymph nodes were dissected and studied; all 21 were clean. Unfortunately, Dr. Strauss tried to preserve as much breast tissue as possible during the lumpectomy, but post-op indicators show inadequate margins. So, I'll be undergoing a second operation within two weeks. Likely it won't be as traumatic an experience as the initial surgery last Thursday. The migraine headache that lasted a day or two was horrific and created havoc with my recovery right after surgery. Today I feel good. I will still have radiation and some form of chemo, but there's a very good chance of cure.

Thank you, one and all, for your calls and emails, prayers and good wishes, flowers, gifts, etc. I cannot adequately express how much it means to me to know you are rooting for my survival and "thrivival." Love, Cheron

Healing takes time, and patience

I eased into the first week of recovery, four days post op. I'd awakened at 5:30 a.m. with a migraine headache that didn't seem to respond to the strong pain medicine prescribed by my surgeon. Bill was planning to return to work that Monday morning, so we started treating my symptoms aggressively: Dilaudid, Bextra, more Dilaudid, Imitrex, Phenergan and a coffee "cocktail" eased the pain and dizziness over the course of two hours. Bill helped me with my drain care before his departure. I relaxed in bed with Thumb-purr nestled at my side.

Long phone conversations with trusted friends, Anne and Julie, bolstered my spirits as the morning wore on. Julie booked a flight to Seattle from eastern Oregon for January 2-4. She was obviously very worried about my health, physical as well as emotional/spiritual. She had already gone on-line to help me locate resources for dealing with pain as well as alternative therapy choices. We had worked together for ten years in a program for children with disabilities. She knew I liked having choices far better than having the course of my life dictated by outside forces. Feeling victimized or powerless just wasn't a comfortable state for either of us.

The numbness and fluid retention in my upper arm was bothersome. When my orthopedist and friend, Dr. Tobin, called from Salem to check on me, I complained that I'd gained this puffy arm and eight pounds in six days. He told me to start exercising. Before Bill arrived home from work I spent 20 minutes on my stationary bike. He helped me shower, wash my hair and change the dressing on my surgery and drain sites. That lifted my spirits and alleviated the body odor that was becoming rather rank.

Friends had started tending to our immediate needs almost before we arrived home from Salem. Dianne was there in short order with a hearty lentil soup. Two days later one of the women in my writers' group came by with a big pot of chicken soup and homemade bread that smelled heavenly. I felt well enough five days post-op to drive myself to the regular Tuesday potluck lunch at Dorle's house, where another friend (also in my writers' group) served butternut squash and pear bisque, accompanied by a colorful array of salads and desserts. On Wednesday evening, after Bill had gone back on the road to resume his work schedule, Mary (also in my writers' group!) invited me to her house next door for a dinner of salmon and fruit salad, and a video movie in front of her crackling, therapeutic fireplace. It soon became obvious I would be well nourished during my "confinement" and I'd have to watch my portions if I didn't want to gain fifty pounds!

I awoke at 6 a.m. on December 9, hearing Bill's voice on the phone in his office adjacent to our bedroom. Our thirty-two-year-old son was calling from Missouri to talk about his marital problems. His relationship had been going rapidly downhill for a year. Now his wife was contemplating separation in which she and the baby would move to their own apartment. We'd known there was high-level stress in their household, but they'd been in counseling attempting to work things out. Attempts were failing. Bill turned the phone over to me. I sat up in bed, taking on my dual role of mom and counselor, listening to my son relate his woes for nearly forty-five minutes until I realized I was growing faint! I did my best to be attentive, but finally had to end the conversation in the interest of self-preservation.

"Oh, Lord, I thought we'd raised our son and given him the tools to overcome the effects of his Asperger's Disorder so he could lead a reasonably normal life despite his autism. We've always contended with his deficits, but expected his strengths would prevail. The social manifestations of the disorder just keep getting worse. Probably a good thing he's in Missouri and not closer. I need to compartmentalize so his issues don't get in the way of my need to focus on beating this cancer. Sounds selfish. But, I need to be healthy and alive if I'm going to be a good mother. Good God, I need you now to help me find the best course of action, and to especially be with this little family that needs your intervention. Help! My head is aching. Better get some coffee and nourishment to go with the aspirin. Looks like I'm up early enough to watch the sun rise over the Cascades. I need inspiration and light badly.

I read my email messages, including a dozen get-well wishes from loved ones all over the country. My Seattle sister, Alice, sent a quote from Upward Bound, a part of the program where she worked at North Seattle Community College. "Don't save anything for a special occasion. Being alive is a special occasion." It was obvious that everyone really wanted me to stay alive and enjoy life a while longer.

My exercise class leader, Doris, called at 10:30 to see

how my recovery was going. "I'm getting along pretty well," I reported. "How is Carl today?" Her reply made me realize I'd been out of the loop. My last class attendance had been on December 1, when I shared the news of my impending surgery with the group. Doris' husband had died of cancer the following day. I'd not been informed so was totally unaware of all she'd been through. But, here she was, calling to ascertain my status and to give her words of encouragement. The compassionate outreach was typical of this little lady. I immediately called Allie to offer my donation to the funds being collected in Carl's memory, which would allow the class to buy memorial stones in the nearby state park.

By Wednesday I was feeling quite well. My self-talk had included a pledge to slow down in order to maximize the healing process, yet to figure out at least one good project a day to keep me distracted from cancer concerns. This day I decided to tie up a loose end by prepping and mailing an appeal for donations to an endowment fund I'd started the year before. I had completed ten years on the national board and three years as president of the American Society for Deaf Children. The endowment project represented my special, ongoing effort to address the organization's constant need for funding to run the non-profit operation. I wrote a letter to encourage donors' holiday spirit of giving and reminding them that a donation now would count as they prepared their income tax forms. When the thirty-five envelopes were all stamped and sealed, I walked several blocks to the mailbox. Feeling rejuvenated by the crisp winter air, I returned home and colored the gray root patches beginning to show in my brunette hair. The effort transformed my "bed hair" into a reasonably attractive coif, which also inspirited me. Done with my mailing project and my hair project, I was content to have completed a productive day. I could relax again. I went to Mary's for dinner and ended up falling asleep on her sofa.

My follow-up appointment with my primary doctor in Port Townsend was encouraging. He affirmed all the decisions we'd made up to that time, and endorsed the oncologists we'd heard about in Bremerton and Sequim. He made the referrals initiating the process to get me scheduled for chemotherapy and radiation. With a second operation to occur in Salem the next week, then Christmas shortly thereafter, we settled on appointments December 29 and 30. Bill rearranged his work schedule and postponed committing to any more jobs until we had a fix on what my needs would dictate. Once these priority dates were on the calendar, I could turn my attentions to the half-dozen other activities I'd planned for the busy holiday month ahead. First, Katie's graduation, December 13…

Relatives are coming from Seattle and at least twenty people have responded to my invitation to attend her party at our house on Saturday. I'm NOT going to let this cancer treatment screw up all the plans we've made…at least I hope not. I feel pretty good, although I've been told to take it easy. Thank goodness for all my friends who are doing most of the cooking for me. I'll make myself take naps during the day. I'll discipline myself to sit and read or write instead of the usual routine of out-and-about activities. Lord, give me patience and help me to be wise. I'm not good at "sedentary."

Ginger knew I was beginning to fret about Katie's party. I hadn't done any housework since before Thanksgiving so the dust and dirt was beginning to show. She arrived at my doorstep before 10 a.m. Friday with an armload of roses, one bouquet for Katie and one for me. Then she set to work vacuuming the entire house from top to bottom. She moved all the furniture and crawled on her hands and knees to be sure all the dirt and pet hair was removed along the baseboards. She joked, "I didn't come to dust your furniture. I hate dusting. You'll have to do that yourself!" Which was certainly within my capacity to handle. The carpet was the cleanest it had been since the weeks after it was installed three years earlier, when we still had two active dogs and a large grey cat shedding their hairy coats year-round.

By 2 p.m. I was headed west to pick up my Seattle sister, Alice, at the ferry terminal. She worked half days on Fridays so planned to come for the long weekend to help out in any way possible. Alice had three boys of her own. Realizing she would never have the girl she desired, she had pledged thirty years earlier to be the best auntie ever, and especially loved doting on all her nieces. Katie's graduation was as important to her as were her own children's achievements. We got back to the house in time to welcome Katie and Ryan, who proceeded to hang pink streamers and balloons from the ceiling beams. The house looked festive, AND very clean. I relaxed in the knowledge that it was going to be a wonderful weekend. Alice and I bundled up to attend holiday open house events at several Victorian bed and breakfast establishments where we treated ourselves to a "dinner" of delectable sweets and wassail.

We headed back to town early Saturday morning for the annual Christmas cookie sale at the Episcopal Church. The line stretched out into the street twenty minutes before opening. These revelers, as those the night before, exuded good cheer and elevated my spirits, even while we pushed and shoved just a little to get to the best looking cookies before they were all gone.

This is the best medicine: being out and about to soak up the abundant comfort and joy of the season. Some friends and neighbors I've encountered seem surprised that I'm not home recovering from surgery. But they're happy to see me smiling and jovial. There is such healing warmth in their greetings and hugs. Life is good...at least it appears far preferable to the alternative right now.

The graduation ceremony for the inaugural class of City University's Master in Teaching program at Port Hadlock, Washington, was a delightful affair. Katie had a rooting section of ten relatives and friends from the Olympic Peninsula and the Seattle area. Afterwards a group of thirty well wishers congregated at our house to fete Katie's accomplishment. The mother of one of her students at the Port Angeles youth center where Katie worked for Americorps had decorated a sheet cake with the symbols of the teaching profession: a ruler border surrounding red apples, books, crayons, a globe, scissors and a blackboard. Bill had purchased a very large pink poinsettia from the Salem Hospital Auxiliary to adorn my hospital room. Now it, along with the white and yellow roses from Ginger, decorated the house with little hint of Christmas. I'd wanted this celebration to be it's own very special event, not mingled with the usual stream of holiday festivities that occur throughout December. By five o'clock the crowd dispersed, leaving an aura of contentment filling our house as it quieted for the start of the winter evening. "Thanks, Mom, it was a wonderful day," Katie said as she hugged me before driving home to Port Angeles.

Mission accomplished! We've enjoyed twenty-four hours of pride and joy without any mention or thought of CANCER. I feel fantastic. Now I have a couple days to clean up and set the house back to rights at a leisurely pace. Must attend to my drain care (yuk), then I can put my feet up for a while. Children's Christmas pageant during worship service tomorrow, and I'll need to pack for the return trip to Salem. Outpatient surgery Thursday afternoon. I'm anxious to have it behind me.

It was an easy decision to not decorate the house or a

tree, having already hosted a party for any family and friends likely to drop by in the coming weeks. There was a good chance no one but Bill and I would be around to see any of it, and putting it up would mean having to take it down. Better to save my energy for quiet healing. Instead, I set up six of my nativity sets, appreciating the slogan, "Jesus is the reason for the season."

Monday afternoon I called to check in with our son. As he bemoaned the facts of his problematic life, I tried to help him assess his plight from a more objective perspective. I encouraged him to avoid wallowing and getting stuck in all the negative baggage he had accumulated. He seemed well aware of his failures but unable to learn from mistakes and formulate plans to move ahead. It wasn't a very rewarding or fruitful conversation, but I felt I'd made an effort to help. The ball was in his court.

Monday evening, while Bill and I watched TV, Santa Claus came to our door. With a jolly "Ho, Ho, Ho" he delivered a lovely red poinsettia plant with a card signed, "Love and get-well wishes, from your Secret Sister." Nearly a year earlier I had co-led our church's annual women's retreat, at which time one of the participants had chosen my name for special attention throughout 2003. I had been showered on several occasions with greeting cards and small, personal gifts to surprise and delight me. Until now the secret had been preserved, but I put two and two together and surmised that my secret sister was married to the man in the red suit standing on my porch. Vince was well known as a jolly old elf that donned the Santa costume to spread cheer throughout the community every holiday season. So, Mary Ann's identity had been revealed! She would continue being attentive throughout the upcoming months, keeping me company during a chemo infusion session, driving me to a radiation treatment, and opening her home to accommodate our friends from Chicago and Oregon who came to visit in July.

Tuesday morning I was grooming and watering my houseplants in preparation for the ensuing trip to Salem. One lovely plant I'd inherited from my mother when she downsized was called "crown of thorns." Its green foliage was dotted with numerous red blooms, year-round; the stems were also covered with sharp thorns. I managed to get a tiny thorn embedded in my left forefinger. My attempts to dig it out with a needle only aggravated the situation, and I thought I could see infection and swelling growing by the minute! Of course, I was overreacting, yet it grew painful and I was mindful of the proscriptions I'd heard about not injuring my left arm and hand because they had been compromised by the surgery and removal of lymph glands. Lacking dexterity with my right, non-dominant hand, I realized I needed help, pronto. Neither Mary nor Dianne, my close-by neighbors, was home, so I called Georgia who lived about a mile away. I figured she'd be sympathetic since she was a breast cancer survivor. She came in short order to extract the sliver and bandage the reddened finger. The whole incident made me feel a little foolish and helpless. Yet, it was indicative of my increased vulnerability and need to depend on others for assistance to help me through the challenges during the cancer treatment months that lay ahead. Indeed, I found scores of people willing and anxious to lend a hand, and I learned to open myself to their healing touch and gestures. It was both humbling and reassuring.

That afternoon Katie drove from Port Angeles, picked me up, then continued to Seattle for the holiday party that Alice and our niece, Tina, had planned at Mom's residence. She now lived in an adult family home where she could get the assistance she needed daily. Alice had created a tradition of gathering all the Seattle-area family members for a soup supper and dessert, making a dinner party, which included all five elderly residents. A number of grandchildren and great-grandchildren brought their liveliness to the affair. All gathered around as the matriarch opened her gifts.

We had decided not to tell Mom about my breast cancer. Her only son had been diagnosed with pancreatic cancer just six years earlier. He died seventeen months later after a valiant battle and a series of painful, experimental treatments. Mom had never recovered from the strain of his long ordeal and his death. The great competence she had always demonstrated began to decline rapidly, until she had to relocate, unable to manage her own home and affairs. She had ceased to read, write, watch TV – most days she preferred lying in her bed all day except for mealtime. Outings, like Katie's graduation party or a Saturday at the stadium to watch the Huskies play college football, were a monumental effort for the family members who accompanied and attended to her. Her awareness of the world was very limited now. She didn't need to know about another child dealing with cancer.

Cut it ALL out!

Bill swung by from his work site north of the city to pick me up for the drive to Salem, four hours away. After a good night's sleep at the motel, I had a list of things to do around town, determined to keep busy until my pre-op appointment with Dr. Strauss late in the day. While Bill saw a full schedule of patients, I took his printer in for repairs at the Apple Store, visited our son's grave with a Christmas bouquet, stopped to see Myrna, our biking buddy, at her counseling center, and visited my former co-workers at the Oregon COPE Project. I spent another hour shopping for bargains at the Grocery Outlet. I still felt energetic and optimistic at the doctor's office. In a nutshell, he reported that the tumor he'd excised was 1.8cms and the lymph nodes were clean. I'd need to keep the drain in place to get through the next phase of recovery, still targeting a goal of no more than 10ccs of drainage per day. The next day he planned to remove a generous section of tissue where lab tests had detected suspicious cells. Back at the motel I walked on the treadmill for a little while, then we cooked TV dinners in the microwave and watched a Jack Nicholson movie and a *Law and Order* re-run to finish the evening. In the midst of all this high stress, I found myself treasuring the simple, mundane activities easing us through to the end of the day.

With surgery scheduled for early afternoon, the morning without food or drink seemed very long. Noel visited me at the surgery center in his role as chaplain. The operation went well and I had no problems waking up and getting mobilized. Bill drove me to the motel to sleep off the remaining sedative in my system. He returned a couple hours later with groceries for his patient: apple juice and saltines to test my digestive system; cheese, chocolate and hot tea at 8 p.m. when we felt assured my stomach could handle it.

After an early appointment on Friday we headed back to Port Townsend, arriving with plenty of time for me to address and stamp one hundred envelopes for our Christmas mailing. Bill helped me create a collage of family pictures we could reproduce with our home computer technology. We chose to highlight Katie's graduation, our toddler grandson's Christmas photo, our summer '03 trip to Prague, and a tiny snapshot of our tom cat, Thumb-purr, who we'd rescued from the shelter earlier in the year. At the very end I added a note about my cancer and surgery. The following week the mail volume was increased dramatically as get-well cards were added to holiday greeting cards. Don, a close friend through our board service for the American Society for Deaf Children, sent an evergreen bouquet with red carnations and candy canes; Darrell, my Peace Corps buddy whose wife had died of breast cancer, sent roses.

I had planned in November, prior to my diagnosis, to

attend the December potluck meeting of the local American Association of University Women chapter, where the Rain-shadow chorale was scheduled to perform. I'd been back and forth to Oregon twice for surgery, yet I wasn't willing to cancel my social outings unless absolutely necessary. Despite the cold weather, the fellowship of these women was warm, the food was delicious, and the music was joyous and uplifting. I found myself sitting in the midst of women I hardly knew, yet felt safe to disclose the news of my illness. Most of them were acquainted with breast cancer survivors. They shared encouraging stories and good wishes. Back home I tucked myself in for a nap with Thumb-purr at my side, getting re-invigorated to complete the Christmas mailing and send out an email report before I retired for the night.

December 21 [email Health Update] *Hallelujah! We're home again and I'm feeling good. A bit of discomfort but no pain (thanks to Vicodin). The second operation at midday last Thursday was far less taxing than the first. Though I know both surgery and cancer are serious subjects, I'm pleased to report that we are relieved and very optimistic about the future. The tumor is all gone; there's nothing to suggest lymph node involvement. They evaluated twenty-one nodes and found NO cancer. I still have the drain in; I am exercising to gain strength and mobility in my left arm (dominant side). My chest is a little lopsided, but gravity will doubtless do some equalizing over time! We have appointments with oncologists closer to home on 12/29 and 12/30. I expect to have chemotherapy, but we don't know what type. There's a good chance it will be oral meds over five years rather than the IV course of treatment that can have so many negative side effects. I'll write again after our upcoming consultations. For now, Christmas blessings to all, dear friends and rellies! Love, Cheron*
    [Mental note: Keep these dispatches informative, but

upbeat. Sharing some of the medical details, as well as emotions, is educational. I want my loved ones to be better informed about breast cancer since it has become so prevalent, but I don't want to induce fear, or pity. Educational but upbeat – that's the ticket!]

Bill and I looked forward to Christmas week with few responsibilities. We'd hunker down at home in front of a fire. Bill was willing to pamper me. We had some leftovers from meals friends had brought. He could warm those or put together easy meals from groceries on hand. One afternoon Dianne showed up bearing a meal of Cornish game hens with all the trimmings, enough for two dinners.

We were very focused on drain care to reduce the discharge so it could be removed. The chance of infection increased every day the drain stayed in place. The output had stabilized between 25ccs and 43ccs per day, a far cry from the 10cc goal. We decided I should discontinue the arm exercises since they exacerbated the drainage problem. We mostly rested, watched TV, and enjoyed phone conversations with well-wishers calling from all over the country. I worked a couple hours every day writing my memoir at the computer.

I surfed the Net trying to find a cocker spaniel needing a home. There were several available on Petfinder.com; one seemed to fit our criteria to a tee. The Peninsula Chapter of Rescue Every Dog (RED) listed an eight-month-old female named Lucy. She had been in foster care with an adoring family for nearly two months, during which time she was treated surgically for a condition called "cherry eye." The vet had surgically corrected the prolapsed gland of the third eyelid. Lucy was spayed, chipped, and current with her shots, housebroken, very loving and non-aggressive. In November we had taken a cocker from a Seattle foster home, on trial, but he turned out to be hyperactive, lifting his leg to mark his territory on our walls and furniture, and determined to catch Thumb-purr for a snack! Undaunted in my love for cocker spaniels, I was ready to try again. Lucy sounded like a winner. I filled out all the forms, assuring RED that we had a fenced area in the yard, a reliable veterinarian and a dog groomer. My concern was that someone else would snatch this opportunity to adopt Lucy ahead of us. Bill seemed as anxious as I to locate a new dog to keep me company while I would be spending more time at home alone.

I found I could use my stationary bike and elliptical trainer for 20-30 minute sessions, to keep my lower body and my heart tuned. However, I was noticing increased lower back pain. We surmised it was from too many hours lying in bed, so I tried napping sitting up in the recliner. It was the back pain that made us decide to skip the Christmas Eve candlelight service at church. We weren't willing to skip out on our invitation to join Mary's family for dinner next door. Among her married children – Cath and Eric, Pat and Beth, Dave and Rene – were many good cooks. Dave grilled savory steaks, the centerpiece for a bounteous holiday table and a five-course dinner accompanied by cheery conversation and the laughter of a loving family coming together to celebrate the season.

Mary gave me a box of See's chocolates passed along from our mutual friend and neighbor, Nellie, who thought I needed the calories more than she did. The three of us had been members of the "Healing After Loss" group at our Presbyterian Church for a year. Nellie and Mary, like most of the group members, were widows who found comfort and healing in sharing the realities of their experience after losing a spouse. I had joined the group because the memoir I was writing detailed my grief work after the death of our little boy, Scotty. That long-ago experience was much in my thoughts, so I believed I could both give and gain insights by being a part of the support group.

Ryan had been assigned duty aboard his Coast Guard

ship for Christmas Eve, so Katie and her greyhound, Lexi, came to spend that night and Christmas Day with her folks. True to form, Katie was very attentive and loving, seemingly content to be back home as the only child for a while. We lounged around the house until mid-afternoon when we went to the historic Rose Theater for a matinee showing of "In America," a heartwarming family movie. It turned out to be a delightful treat. Bill and I hadn't been to a movie with one of our children for many years, and especially not in the middle of the day, or on Christmas.

Sister Alice and her husband came from Seattle to Port Townsend on Friday evening. Bill and I had developed a Christmas tradition of giving them a gift certificate for a weekend at a Port Townsend bed and breakfast. Besides the enjoyment of their visit, it was a way to thank Alice for her extraordinary efforts in support of our aging mother. This year the couple was using the gift immediately in order to share a part of the holidays with us. They settled into the Commander's Beach House, and then called to plan our time together. My lower back pain was limiting my mobility, despite painkillers, so we planned to get together the following afternoon.

Just when I've begun feeling relieved that the tumor was removed from my body, this back pain causes suspicion about possible metastasis. Can the cancer cells have found their way into my spine? Perish the thought! Guess that's something we can investigate when we see the oncologist in Bremerton on Monday. Three days from now...I'll try to avoid worrying. Get my attitude right! The backache is probably totally unrelated to the cancer. Three days to relax and enjoy the relatives visiting all weekend.

Alice and her Bill went kayaking Saturday morning, arriving at our house in time to watch the televised game between the Seahawks and the Forty-niners. Hawks won!

Because December 29 was our thirty-sixth anniversary, Bill and Alice treated us to dinner at the Ajax Café. They left Sunday morning, but soon thereafter Alice's son, David, arrived with his family for a visit and work session. We adopted David as our computer guru. He'd developed this expertise as engineer for the community college television project. This day we'd hired (bribed) him to spend a day helping us refine our computer hardware and software. We shared a pizza lunch, thoroughly enjoying the antics of David's five-year-old daughter as she played in our house and yard.

Our consultation with Dr. Ann Murphy at the Olympic Hematology and Oncology Program was very helpful. Her manner was personable; she answered all our questions about treatment options. We came away convinced that I should undergo the full regimen of chemo, radiation and follow-up oral hormones. Her comment: "There's a good chance that, if you choose to have all the treatment forms, and you continue to lead a healthy lifestyle with diet and exercise, you might expect to live your normal life expectancy of eighty-five years." That prognosis was pretty convincing.

Our day in Bremerton helped us to plan for the rigors of the months ahead. If all proceeded according to expectations, I would complete the aggressive protocols before the end of June. I'd start with chemotherapy, four infusion treatments spaced twenty-one days apart. We viewed the large room where a dozen patients were undergoing chemotherapy that afternoon. Some of these folks appeared very ill while others looked healthy except for their IVs or injection apparatuses. We learned I'd be getting a chemo "cocktail" of two drugs commonly used for breast cancer patients: Adriamycin and Cytoxan. I would be provided with heavy doses of anti-nausea medication. Some would be injected or infused, but other doses could be administered by mouth or anal suppository. Dr. Murphy and her cadre of nurses assured us that science had come a long way in the treatment of nausea and other chemo side effects. I WOULD lose all of my hair, very likely within the first two weeks after the initial infusion.

We negotiated with the doctor to schedule my first treatment on Monday, January 19. This would allow us to take a trip to Palm Springs that we'd been planning since fall. There was an orthopedic training conference Bill planned to attend there. We would be staying with good friends, Don and Carol, who'd been very attentive since learning of my diagnosis. They could be counted upon to pamper me during the visit extending from January 10 to January 17. Seeing them and soaking up the southern California sun would be good therapy. In the meantime, I'd need to return to Bremerton on both January 6 and January 8 for pre-chemo tests. One, called a "MUGA," was a radiology test to check my heart strength. The other would be a total body bone scan to be sure my back and joint pain, as well as depressed white blood count, were not related to cancer. I was told to monitor the drainage from my surgical site and do whatever possible to decrease the volume of secretions. They would not be able to begin chemo on January 19 if the drain were not removed by then.

"Lucy, I'm home!" – Ricky Ricardo

As we crossed the Hood Canal Bridge returning home to Pt. Townsend, Bill's cell phone rang with a call from the foster mom for Lucy, the cocker spaniel. She apologized for the delay in responding to my application, but invited us to come meet the dog anytime. Linda and her husband lived within ten miles of the Bremerton clinic where we spent the afternoon. So, we turned the car around at the end of the bridge and headed back. It was love at first sight! Lively Lucy had a soft, cinnamon-colored coat and beautiful brown eyes. She wiggled and danced joyfully in her desire to get acquainted, up close and personal. She crawled into our laps and showered us with dog kisses. Linda filled us in regarding the dog's idiosyncrasies, all of which seemed perfectly dog-like and charming to us. She related how Lucy's original owner had named her after the redheaded comedienne, Lucille Ball, so that he could come in the door after work each evening and call out in the accent of Ricky Ricardo, "Lucy, I'm home!" RED required a home-visit before any adoption could be completed, so we arranged for Linda to check out our canine accommodations in Port Townsend two days later.

This really tickles me. Bill is every bit as excited about adopting Lucy as I am. Cockers have always been my favorite breeds, ever since we had cocker mixes in my childhood home. I best remember Lucky, a black and brown female who blessed us with three litters of puppies in less than two years – twenty-four puppies in total. We found good homes for all of them. Robinhood, the party-colored cocker I found at the shelter in Salem, was a part of our family for several years in the '90s. Bill teased me incessantly about "Robbie's" sweet nature, and yet how dumb he was. He never mastered housebreaking, and he tended to slam into walls racing around inside the house. Always happy-go-lucky, he'd recover quickly from the collision to go merrily on his way. Robbie was a jewel compared to the very trying week we'd spent with the cocker who was on a mission to kill Thumb-purr! Let bygones be bygones...Lucy appears to be a blessing. Thank God Linda caught up with us today. I can hardly wait to welcome Lucy on New Year's Eve.

Early Tuesday morning we drove thirty miles in the opposite direction for consultation at the Cancer Center in Sequim. Dr. Clare Bertucio, the radiation oncologist, took a thorough history and examination, remarking that the site where the drain exited my underarm showed signs of potential infection. There were many negative side effects that might occur from the radiotherapy, all of which were carefully explained. I was glad to have Bill listening and evaluating the risks, using his expertise to judge the potential benefits. In his opinion, they definitely outweighed the risks. We were told there would be a couple days of testing and preparation in Sequim prior to initiation of radiation therapy. The therapy itself would consist of thirty-three treatments that would occur five days a week for six and a half weeks as long as I didn't develop any contraindications, like skin, lung or heart damage. We were instructed to schedule appointments there as soon as we could estimate the date for completion of chemotherapy.

On the return trip home I consulted my calendar to see if this therapy regimen was going to conflict with any of the activities we'd planned for 2004. I was relieved that we'd not have to cancel the Palm Springs trip. I'd been planning to surprise all my friends on the board of the American Society for Deaf Children (ASDC) when they gathered from all over the nation for a meeting in the Portland area in late March. Then I remembered my 40th college reunion was to occur in late June. I was going to be bald in March and June! I called this to Bill's attention. He replied, "Honey, just order a great wig and go as a blonde bombshell!" Sounded like fun.

Then there was the trip we'd planned to bike the Katy Trail across Missouri with Noel and Myrna the end of April. We decided not to cancel that, either, unless it became apparent that I wouldn't have the strength and stamina. That biking trek would fit nicely in the space between my last chemo infusion and the beginning of daily radiation in May. In August we'd planned to take Katie on a European river cruise as a graduation gift. Being desperately interested in seeing the world, I only hoped I'd be healthy and strong for that adventure. Bill said, "We'll play it by ear and go with the flow." He'd prioritized his life and work schedules to spend as much time with me as was necessary.

Hooray! It's Lucy day. I hope our home will pass inspection so Lucy can be a part of our family from the very start of the new year. I feel almost as much excitement as when we brought home our new babies from the hospital. Actually, adopting Lucy into our lives will probably be lots easier. She's supposed to be a "sack hound" that loves to sleep late and doesn't wake in the night. She returns your affection tenfold, and she poops outside.

Linda called offering to stop by PetCo to buy a harness and an ID tag for Lucy. I was waiting at the window when they pulled into our driveway. Lucy emerged in the arms of Linda's daughter, who was having some separation anxiety. We all watched as Lucy piddled a little in the front hallway. We were used to cockers' "excited utterances," as Bill called them. She took off on a wild chase when she saw Thumb-purr, obviously wanting to play, not harm. The cat raced through the pet door leading to the fenced dog run. Lucy stopped short, but coaxing and teaching only a few times introduced her to this channel for independent exit and entrance. The premises passed inspection so we signed on the dotted line and paid the adoption fee, making Lucy a bona fide Mayhall! That night Thumb-purr kept his distance while Lucy cuddled in our big bed as if she'd been sleeping there forever. It would be some weeks before the canine-feline friendship developed enough for them to settle in as bed partners. Linda asked that we keep in touch by email and offered to dog-sit whenever Lucy needed a place to stay while we traveled. We told them about the week we planned to be in Palm Springs. They scheduled Lucy's "hotel" reservation on their calendar!

A new year begins

It's feeling like a Happy New Year, even if I can't stay awake for fireworks or the ball to drop in Times Square. Lucy's here. We know pretty much what's in store for us between now and June. Blocking the activities into a calendar helps me to feel more in control, less like a victim. Lord, I'm thankful for Bill's love and attention. Bless him and all the friends and family members who are coming out of the woodwork to offer their support. They help me to feel confident and strong.

Julie called early on January 2 to tell me her flight had been cancelled. She had driven through the snow from her rural home in northeastern Oregon to the Tri-cities airport in Washington. Weather conditions over the Cascade Mountains were stormy, grounding most flights into Seattle. I assured her I'd be fine, but not before scheduling a rain check visit after the thaw. She and her husband, Peter, would drive to Port Townsend for a weekend in the spring.

I wrote an email update to my cyber support group, now numbering 40: Saturday, January 3:

About twenty years ago there was a spate of sci-fi TV programs and a movie or two featuring bald women in starring roles, i.e. Sigourney Weaver. I remember wondering at the time how I would look bald. Now I'm going to have an opportunity to find out. Bill and I will probably have matching hairstyles by Valentine's Day, and I'll be in the billiard-ball category for the advent of spring!

We spent the early part of last week with oncologists in Bremerton and Sequim, communities within fifty miles and thirty miles of our house, respectively. I am set up for a couple of tests – complete body bone scan and MUGA (heart strength related) – this next week in Bremerton.

These are part of the pre-chemo work-up. If all goes well, I will begin the series of four chemotherapy treatments, spaced 21 days apart, on January 19. In the interim, Bill and I will escape for a week to Palm Springs and sunshine. We planned this trip in September, an opportunity for Bill to earn continuing education credits, and a visit with friends there to keep me entertained. Should be a good respite before an intense six months of treatments.

If there are no complications, my chemo will be over by mid-April. I'll get a little break, then start daily trips to Sequim for 6-8 weeks in May and June. Evidently the radiation usually doesn't make the patient sick, so I will be able to do this back-and-forth driving on my own. Our good friends, Anne and Hans, live in Sequim, so there'll be occasions for lots of visits with them.

After radiation, I will be on oral hormonal therapy for about five years. Hopefully that'll take care of it and I'll not have to worry about more cancer arising. The oncologist in Bremerton impressed us with her knowledge and manner. We are comfortable following her recommendations for all of this. She says that this aggressive approach makes sense since I am young and otherwise healthy. Our goal is to get me back to the probability of living out my full life expectancy, another 25 years or so. Sounds good to me!

Please keep us in your thoughts and prayers as this odyssey unfolds. I will check in from time to time to let you know how it's going. In addition to all of you cyber-supporters, we have a wonderful local support network. Many good friends through Habitat, church and neighborhood here in Port Townsend, and family members just "across the pond" in Seattle. People are signing up to bring food so I don't have to cook after chemo treatments. I have no doubt we'll be well-fed and struggling to keep from getting roly-poly as well as bald!

I'm planning to go to my 40th college reunion at Pacific

University in late June. If I don't have a satisfactory crop of new hair, Bill says I should buy a glamorous wig and go as a blonde bombshell. Sounds like a great way to keep our sense of humor through all of this.

Wishing you all a healthy and happy new year. Love, Cheron and Bill

Writer's group met the first Monday in January. I hadn't made much progress on "The Bridge Is Love," my memoir/novel, but my creative writing friends were just glad I was well enough to be with them. They were interested to hear about my "cancer journey" and offered support. Mary, Evelyn, Dusty, Beth and Willean were becoming some of my closest friends as we shared our lives and entrusted our attempts at artistic expression to each other's critiques. I found myself making a mental list of all the women who were volunteering some of their precious time to help me through my crisis. I knew I could count on all five of this group.

I determined to take stock of my life in an attempt to streamline my activities, making a list of all my commitments as well as the special events I hoped to enjoy or tasks that would require time and energy. I needed to simplify and prioritize.

1. Writers' Group – one morning meeting a month, supplying encouragement for my desire to write. Try to continue writing an average of ten hours each week.

I suppose it's going to be harder to commit blocks of time to writing, not knowing if and when I'll feel up to it. I'll make an effort to drop less important activities so I can write when I'm asymptomatic. Maybe I can use the cancer as an incentive...a reason to focus and persist. I'm writing "The Bridge" because it's an important story to share. If *my life is going to be shorter or my health diminished, more than I'd previously thought, I <u>must</u> keep working to complete my manuscript. If I don't write this book, the tale will never be told.*

2. Trustees – one evening meeting per month and assorted interim, volunteer activities. I knew this trusty church group would rather have my service be irregular than for me to resign.
3. Healing After Loss group – Again, I could play this one by ear and go only when I had plenty of time and energy.
4. American Association of University Women – I'd signed up for a hiking group and the scholarship committee. This was a large and thriving group that could function well without me!
5. Women's retreat planning committee – I kept the March weekend event on my calendar and let the planners know to call me if I was needed for anything else.
6. Worship and Theology Committee for the Presbytery – One, hour-long meeting in Seattle per month, with two hours of travel time on each end. Five more hours I should save for healing and writing. I contacted the chairman to request a leave of absence.
7. Neighborhood exercise group – Two or three, hour-long sessions a week at a location just five minutes from our house. I'd go whenever I could, for the social contact as much as the physical workout.
8. Curves for Women – My Tues/Thurs/Sat workout opportunity in town. My annual membership was due to expire. I'd "cool my jets" and take a medical leave until I completed my treatment.
9. El Salvador mission liaison – I had the experience and expertise to facilitate the planning for the group

traveling to Central America in August. It was unlikely I'd be going, but I could use my computer and telephone from home to set up flight and lodging schedules and I could teach the group some basic Spanish before their departure in late summer.

10. PLASDC (Past Leaders of the American Society for Deaf Children) – This was my baby to nurture, an endowment fund I'd set up after my presidency with this national group. I could still send out the forty, semi-annual letters appealing for donations. The task was to be assumed by another person in 2005. I needed to keep it going until then.

11. Tuesdays with Dorle luncheons – A must! I might not feel like a hearty lunch and lots of company the Tuesdays after Monday chemo treatments, but other Tuesdays, YES!

12. Habitat for Humanity – Ginger and I had decided to withdraw as sponsors for the family currently building their house, with hopes for assuming that role with a future family. As for my shifts working at the re-sale store, I'd continue with that twice a month on non-chemo weeks. These fellow volunteers were important members of my support system and they'd understand if I sat down on the job or worked a shorter shift than the rest.

13. Get-togethers with my high school "gal pals" in Seattle -- not to be missed! One of them was a recent breast cancer survivor. All of them humored me and bolstered my spirits.

14. Availability to support Bill's work and his service on the neighborhood association board of directors. He'd manage these just fine without me for a while.

15. Learn how to groom Lucy. At-home haircuts, once a month, can do!

16. Yard work as spring arrives – I determined not to get stressed about it.

Though the list seemed long, many of the activities were infrequent and my absences, as necessary, wouldn't create problems. In fact, I realized I might not even be missed because life goes on and others take up the slack. I wasn't indispensable; my most important task was to focus on healing.

I refused to cancel any of the trips on our events calendar: Palm Springs in January, ASDC meeting in Portland the end of March, biking trip across Missouri on the Katy Trail in April, followed by a weekend in San Diego for Bill's medical conference, my 40th college reunion in late June, and our graduation-gift trip with Katie to cruise and bike in Europe during August.

I need the special events as joys to look forward to, and the busy-ness at home and in the community to normalize our lives. Twenty-four hours in every day that need to be filled with something worthwhile. I'll listen to my body and follow my doctors' advice, but life DOES go on. I'll keep pace as best I can.

Sara responded to my email update of January 3:

Hi Cheron: Good to get your update and to know your humor is intact! Don't concern yourself about the Habitat family you were to partner with. We have found another person to sponsor. Concentrate on YOU and you'll know when you're ready for Habitat again. Since you are going to be doing chemo I wanted to write a little about my experience. I have a wonderful oncologist and have found that most doctors and nurses who deal with cancer are incredible. I'm grateful for their special talents. Rule #1: Do not allow people to tell you horror stories about chemo. I've learned there are over 100 types of chemo and, unless you are taking the same drug, same dosage for the same problem, you're really not getting information that pertains to you. Rule #2: Empower yourself. This is not debilitating. My doctor says there are many powerful women who drive themselves to chemo on Friday at noon, do the treatment, drive themselves home and show up for work on Monday or Tuesday of the following week. The drugs that you get before chemo allow your body to tolerate the toxins. I actually felt very normal. Granted, I was NOT normal, but I felt okay. When I took adriamycin and cytoxan I could have been very nauseated, but I took three different types of anti-nausea medicine and only threw up three times, and that was when I woke up and went too long between medication. I ate normally and, after the fourth or fifth day, started walking again at H.J. Carroll Park. Do not think you can't exercise. You might not be able or want to do as much as normal, but you can certainly adjust it to your ability at the time. Rule #3: Concentrate on you and take good care of yourself. There is no one more important than you during this process. You can say no to people and not feel guilty and you can also do what best suits you. Because I had a somewhat difficult time dealing with people I knew casually, I let Ed do the errands to the grocery store, post office and bank, but I would let him take me out to dinner at Ajax Café (I wore a great hat) and a seafood place we found in downtown Poulsbo.

I certainly wouldn't wish that anyone go through chemo, but (this will be hard to understand) it was the best thing that ever happened to me. Take a deep breath here. I live my days feeling like a totally different person. I feel so much joy each and every day and only concentrate on the good in my life. Yeah, I still have to clean the toilet and change the sheets, but I'm living life on my own terms. If I want to do something, I do it. I exercise about five times a week and that also helps me feeling so healthy!!! I value the friends that I have and appreciate the little things in life...I could go on and on. I've been given a second chance that I am truly grateful for and I have no plans to screw it up this time. Please let me know if you have questions I might help you with. You are in my prayers each night. Love, Sara

This very welcome pep talk infused new courage into my soul on January 5th. I didn't then know that I was about to begin the ten most distressful and frustrating days of the whole six-month treatment process. The next day I started what felt like a ride on an out-of-control roller coaster. There were ups and downs and hills and valleys to seriously try my patience and dampen my humor and optimism.

I went to bed on January 5th almost anticipating the MUGA test of my heart muscle the following day. Lucy and I arose early for the drive to Bremerton and were almost ready to depart when the phone rang. A winter storm had hit particularly hard thirty miles south of us, closing roads and medical offices. My test had to be rescheduled for two days later. It could be performed instead of the bone scan scheduled on Thursday. The bone scan was postponed until the day of my first chemo treatment, January 19. The beauty of the falling snow outside our door, which normally would have delighted me, served only slightly to assuage my disappointment for this delay.

I DO get rigid about appointments and scheduling. Once it's on the calendar, I hate being deterred. My mother instilled in us that "...neither rain nor snow nor dark of night shall deter us..." mentality. Okay, this is not my decision. It's out of my control. Blame it on Mother Nature. Pray for clearing weather so the trip to Bremerton on Thursday will be possible. We should be able to catch our scheduled flight to Palm Springs on Saturday.

Relax and enjoy a warm fire. Play with Lucy. She is such a joy, barking hysterically when she sees Thumb-purr. Cat's not intimidated in the least, so the chase behavior

will probably subside shortly. Appreciate the beauty of winter. Don't ruin it by being crabby!

Most of the snow had melted by the next morning. Dianne walked down the block with a pot of lentil soup for our lunch. She was anxious to meet Lucy. Bill was off work for the day. He shared with her some newfound wisdom he'd discovered about computer hardware, software and the Internet. Shortly after her departure I got an email message from an Oregon friend, Darlene. She'd heard through the grapevine about my cancer. Her treatment for breast cancer three years earlier was almost identical to what was being prescribed for me. She confirmed that she'd lost all her hair but it grew back thicker than before the cancer. She'd preferred wearing baseball caps to wigs. Darlene was one of my friends through connections arising out of support for our deaf daughter's needs. She was beautiful and smart, and a published author. She was also deaf. An inspiration in the past, and now a member of the new sisterhood connection I was making because of the cancer.

Progress toward wellness, one step at a time

That evening I attained the goal that allowed for removal of the drainage tube I'd been fussing with for 33 days. Bill snipped a couple of sutures around the exit site, slid the rubber tubing easily out of the wound near my underarm, and freed me from bondage. I hopped into the shower and enjoyed soaping and scrubbing my whole body vigorously without fear of pulling loose that tiresome rubber appendage.

Geeze, it's like getting a ball and chain removed! Whee! I feel free, and CLEAN, really clean. This whole ordeal certainly makes one grateful for the small pleasures and successes in life. One more hurdle out of the way so I get can on with the initiation of chemo treatments next Monday. Hallelujah! Thank you, God.

Removal of the drainage apparatus also facilitated a return to normalcy in our sex life. Thus unencumbered, my body felt free and more agile. Throughout the following months of therapy, our intimacy was unaffected except during the initial week after each of the four chemo infusions, when lethargy and assorted negative symptoms arose. In fact, I felt good about my body as I slowly shed ten excess pounds and dropped a clothing size. This made sexual activity more desirable for me, even though I was bald, and turbaned at night!

The roads were dry and the MUGA test went well on Thursday. The technician who injected the dye and scanned my heart was very pleasant. I passed with flying colors – "75 percent ejection fraction" I was told. This sounded pretty technical and a detail I probably didn't need to understand, as long as I'd passed the test. Afterwards I went by Dr. Murphy's office for the results of my blood work-up. My dreams of the week in sunny Palm Springs quickly faded into disappointment when she told me my white blood cell (WBC) count was very low. She would not okay the start of chemo until she could figure out the cause of my depressed WBC. These infection-fighting cells would decrease markedly and predictably when chemo started, so they needed to be more abundant when the treatments commenced.

I would need a bone marrow test, and that was normally done after the total body bone scan. I was looking at a serious delay in scheduling and I was not a happy patient!

Since the marrow test could not be done on a Friday, the only way to secure the possibility of starting chemo on January 19 was to cancel Palm Springs so we'd be available during that week for the testing. I was disgruntled and disturbed on the drive home, my anger tempered only by the companionship of Lucy and snacking on Cheetos and chocolate bridge mix!

The minute we arrived home I called Bill to share my disappointment and frustration. We decided immediately that getting the tests done and chemo underway was far more important that the trip and his medical conference. Dr. Murphy needed an historical record of my blood tests over the years to establish a baseline for my red and white cell counts. While I called doctors in Pt. Townsend and Salem to glean these from my medical records and fax them to us, Bill contacted Dr. Murphy's office to schedule the two remaining tests as soon as possible. The scan would be on Monday and the bone marrow test on Tuesday of our Palm Springs week. I called Don and Carol in Palm Springs to say we'd not be coming, holding back tears until I hung up the phone. I called Linda to say we'd not be boarding Lucy with her for the week. Both of us cried tears of disappointment.

Julie sent a long email to express some of the thoughts she'd hoped to be sharing face to face. She thanked me for having believed in her during a period when her life was in turmoil and she felt overwhelmed with challenges. I had hired her to work in the project I directed in Oregon to assist families raising children with disabilities.

"You continue to be such a strong influence on my life and my work," she wrote. "Setting up my own counseling practice this past year, I have tried to follow your example as closely as possible. I was looking forward to being there with you as much for consultation as anything – I figured we'd only want to talk about breast cancer part of the time! I have thought of you so often, and the humane but business-like model you developed for handling your staff, always giving people the benefit of the doubt.

"I can't imagine the journey you are on, though I know it is a sacred one, examining the territory between life and death. A couple years ago I read a book inspired by the sudden death of my father-in-law who died of a brain tumor in his mid-60s. It was titled, *One Year to Live,* by Steven Levine. He is a grief therapist who spent 40 years treating terminally ill patients. His book is meant to teach people how to truly live, because so many of us don't live life meaningfully and truly until we face the possibility of death, which inspires us to reevaluate and pare down to essentials. His book helps readers examine their lives, then create lives that fit their hopes and intentions.

"I hope your kids are handling this, especially Phillip so far away and going through his own turmoil. We'll stay in touch and have lots to talk about when Peter and I get to your place in March. I'm determined to live my own life more fully, less work and more time for my creative self and my friendships. That includes you, dear friend. I can't wait to see you. Love, Julie."

While the tech was injecting dye for my scan on Monday, Bill took reports from my blood work during recent years to Dr. Murphy. They demonstrated a consistent pattern of lower-than-normal white cell counts, which made the current results less shocking by contrast. Bill mentioned to the doctor that my back pain continued to be problematic, so they decided to order additional x-rays of my lower spine. Later that afternoon the various x-rays were mounted on the light box for study. They showed "hot spots" in my skeletal shoulder and knee joints, as well as in my lower back. Bill and the radiologist diagnosed plenty of osteoarthritis and scoliosis, but NO signs of bone cancer. Truly good news.

But, I thought the determination of no metastasis was definitive when they studied the 21 excised lymph nodes. All this time I've been feeling confident that surgery had removed ALL the cancer. Take a deep breath; you've passed another hurdle with a declaration of tumor-free bones. Except for the marrow. Damn, I could still have cancer IN-SIDE my bones screwing up the production of my blood cells. We'll be back to get that checked out tomorrow morning. I just want to get chemo underway next week. Please, God, give me patience and move this process along as fast as possible. At least Bill has all this week off since he was supposed to have been in California, so he and Lucy are close by to comfort and support me through these aggravating days.

The nurse practitioner that extracted several vials of marrow from my pelvic bone was a pro. She positioned me in a bent-from-the-waist posture, steadying me in this pose, leaning my body hard against my forearms braced on the wall. Then she rolled up her sleeves, took off her shoes, planted her legs firmly on either side of mine, and set to work tugging and pulling with all her might on the plunger of the large hypodermic needle. It obviously took muscle; she broke a sweat. It was ungraceful and would have appeared lewd to an onlooker who couldn't fathom what was going on!

She explained each step of the procedure, interspersed with chat about family and personal topics to pass the time and lower my anxiety. She also drew more blood samples, the whole process taking only an hour. "It's a real plus that you're not carrying much excess fat on your buttocks," she explained. "It makes getting this large syringe needle through the tissue and into the bone much easier." The pain after the procedure was negligible. The lab report would be delayed one day because the marrow samples had to be sent to Seattle for evaluation.

We decided to pass the time by following a suggestion from the oncology nurse to check out a program that loaned wigs to bald chemo patients. The primary instructor for the cosmetology program at a Bremerton technical college was a breast cancer survivor. She had developed the loaner program, making a community service project part of beautician training. There was a roomful of wigs on Styrofoam heads, every color and style imaginable. I was invited to choose six or eight for starters. Having taken a liking to the "blonde bombshell" idea, I chose seven wigs with yellow-gold tones, plain and frosted, curly and straight, short and long. I grabbed a couple with red and auburn hues, but spurned the grays entirely. I'd been dyeing my gray roots to maintain my brunette hair color for years, and I wasn't ready to succumb to gray until I had a few more grandchildren.

This experience was a hoot! All the young students gathered around to give their opinions, while Bill sat nearby alternately chuckling or shaking his head in amazement. I found myself laughing out loud, something I'd not done much in recent days. One of the curly red wigs was a long Afro style that made me think of Clarabell the Clown from the Howdy Doody television show I'd watched as a child. I liked all but one of the blonde styles and the auburn "Prince Valiant" was an interesting alternative. I garnered many compliments and began to feel pretty, and a little silly, too. They brought a couple of large hatboxes into which they packed eight wigs and the tools and potions to style them, plus several head coverings for day and night wear. Two were in the bandeau-turban style, close fitting and soft, to wear while sleeping. The stylist told me that my bald head would get cold and I'd lose a lot of heat through my scalp during the winter nights. I put one on and sneered at myself in the mirror, wide-eyed. I told my audience that I was impersonating Gloria Swanson's Norma Desmond character in "Sunset Boulevard." None of the youngsters had a clue that the 1940s Hollywood diva looked something like the turbaned princess in the modern Disney Aladdin movie, only older and scarier.

Back home I made dinner while Bill called the airline

for last-minute seats available to Palm Springs. His search paid of. He reserved space on Wednesday evening so he could attend the two final days of his conference and we could have some fun with our southern California friends on the weekend, just prior to chemotherapy session #1. Katie picked up Lucy to dog-sit at her Pt. Angeles apartment while we were away. As we drove to the airport the doctor called Bill's cell phone with the bone marrow results, which were within normal limits. No more delays. The sense of relief was almost palpable as we grinned broadly at one another. The next step in the treatment regimen would commence as scheduled!

I feel really happy and grateful to have my life back on track, leaving the dreary Northwest weather behind for a few days to bask in sunshine. Sara told me about "good days" and "bad days"… "Expect them to balance out." I've been depressed and frustrated some of the time, but also elated and happily relieved when something raises me out of my sorrow. I know both Dianne and Julie have worried about my fears of death. Such thoughts have been fleeting. I'm not entertaining that possibility, much. I keep reminding myself that breast cancer is highly curable with proper treatment. I don't feel my body is sick, and neither is my spirit. This is just another major life challenge for Bill and me, but we've traveled through many valleys together and we're still strong!

I DID recall a discussion that occurred three years earlier at my 40th high school reunion. Jeff, a Seattle lawyer who'd been a friend since kindergarten, calculated the number and percentage of our peers who wouldn't be around for a 50th reunion in 2010. He was advocating for a 45th get-together rather than waiting the usual ten years. The predictable death rate was jarring but, of course, I considered losing only <u>others</u>, like our deceased friends Colin,

Shelley, Steve, Doug, Lila...not me! Now the possibility of dying before 2010 seemed all too real. I tried to squelch the thought. My only grandchild was not yet two years old and I'd expected to see him and our other progeny among his peers graduate and marry. The quote from the statuette Allie had given me – "Life is worth fighting for" – popped into my consciousness. I convinced myself to confront this challenge... one day at a time and never lose hope. Dr. Murphy had predicted my longevity to age 85. Grandson Jeremy might even be a college grad by then!

Sunny days, healing toxins, friends galore

Palm Springs weather was sunny, 70 degrees, flowers blooming abundantly in the neighborhood and a light dusting of snow topping the mountains in the distance. I joined our hosts and their toy poodle, Jed, for a brisk walk each morning. One afternoon I observed as Don groomed Jed, giving me pointers for when I started grooming Lucy at home. We had cocktails and ate dinner with our hosts' neighbors and relatives, then strolled through the street fair booths during the cool evening. We were joined on Saturday by my friend from Peace Corps days, Darrell, who drove to Palm Springs from his hometown about an hour away. Because he'd lost his wife to breast cancer, he knew what these upcoming months of treatment would be like. He was very supportive and encouraging. We went for "early bird" dining at a favorite local restaurant where a duo was performing easy-listening music. The famous Hollywood director, Steven Spielberg, and his party were seated just a few tables away!

We flew home Saturday night, feeling grateful for the respite time away. Katie and Ryan brought Lucy home from Pt. Angeles. In our absence, the pup's "cherry eye" condition had recurred. Ryan had thoroughly enjoyed the playfulness of this small, adorable dog, which contrasted with the demeanor of Katie's more sedate greyhound, Lexi. However, they'd found Lucy's ghoulish, blood-red eye creepy and joked about the "demon cocker spaniel." We'd have to get her to the veterinary ophthalmologist for surgery as soon as possible.

Alice and her son, Danny, came from Seattle early on Sunday to spend the day. Katie joined us and we all attended church together, where the pastor preached a sermon on patience and trusting in God's timing, which often seems too slow. It seemed he was talking most directly to me sitting there in the pew with my family support group.

As soon as Alice had learned my schedule for chemotherapy every third Monday, she arranged her life so she could spend the preceding weekends at our house to help me prepare. For this first expedition of cheer they brought a warm, fleece, hooded bathrobe with a matching lap blanket and slippers. It was red and decorated with Scotty dogs. Danny selected a gift of warm socks decorated with orange cats like Thumb-purr, knowing my fondness for silly socks and sharing my love of cats. Their presence and gifts worked as an encouraging tonic to uplift my spirits as I anticipated the toxic treatments ahead of me.

My excitement and anticipation is so intense you'd think I was going to my wedding rather than to my inaugural chemotherapy treatment! I'm so relieved to be finally getting the infusion phase underway after the uncertainty and delay leading up to this day. I'm not very virtuous in terms of patience when it comes to health care. I can hardly wait for those chemicals to start tracking down and eliminating potential cancer cells throughout my body. Let the games begin!

On January 19, Bill drove Lucy and me to the treatment center 90 minutes away. I had been scoping out the businesses along the route with every intention of using these outings to bargain-shop at some favorite stores we didn't have in our small town: Big Lots, Grocery Outlet, Home Depot and PetSmart. By 10 a.m. I was seated in a comfortable recliner and ready for the nurses to get to work on me. The large room contained a dozen easy chairs for patients, arranged in an arc around the nurses' station. One wall was filled with large windows that let in sunshine, at least on those rare winter days when the rays broke through the clouds on the Kitsap Peninsula. There were also comfortable chairs for friends or family members who accompanied patients and chose to wait during the chemo sessions, which usually lasted several hours. The next day I summarized the experience in my email update to a list that had grown to almost 50 names, with the additions of friends who had contacted me after hearing through the grapevine about my cancer.

Hi All: Yesterday we got back on schedule with my first chemo treatment at the oncology center in Bremerton. It all went well and I'm feeling pretty good now, about 20 hours later. The nurses loaded me up with all kinds of chemicals, both IV infusion and oral meds to bring back home. These should dispel the side effects of nausea that might occur over the next few days.

Some of you know we had a bit of a setback last week and had to delay our vacation to Palm Springs in order to get some additional tests before they'd proceed with the chemo. My heart-strength test was very good. My total body bone scan, followed by some x-ray close-ups of my lumbar spine, showed only osteoarthritis and scoliosis, not cancer. Likewise, the bone marrow test came back okay, although Dr. Murphy says I seem to make about 40 percent fewer white cells than most people. It looks like everything else is functioning as it should. I will have my blood drawn tomorrow and weekly to be sure this low white count isn't a problem as the chemical pervading my system begin to strain my natural defenses.

Bill and I finally did get away for a short, relaxing visit in southern California, and my sister came on Sunday with a retinue of relatives bearing gifts to help me pamper myself on those post-chemo days when I need to stay home to rest in cozy comfort.

So, yesterday we loaded up the new Cocker puppy, Lucy, and headed for the treatment center early. This dog is a great car traveler and will be a fabulous companion as I go hither and yon for treatments during the coming six months. She also keeps Bill busy while I'm sitting in the recliner getting my chemo.

It took four of the nursing staff to find a vein that would work on my right hand/arm. The left is no longer an option since that's the side of my surgery and my lymph system has been compromised. So, they got lots of practice and insight for the next go-round. After the needle was finally in, they started by infusing me with anti-nausea meds. Next the nurse brought a large syringe of red Adriamycin that she eased into my vein manually. This is the chemical responsible for hair loss. That was followed by a large drip bag of Cytoxan. Then, a bag of sterile water to flush it all through. I'm two pounds heavier this morning and I blame it on all that fluid! The reason it is imperative that they get a good vein has mostly to do with the Adriamycin because if any of it leaks out it can cause serious adverse reactions to the skin at the injection site. I appreciate their efforts to find a good blood vessel.

We left with four additional anti-nausea meds, most of which I must take during these three days subsequent to the treatment. If they work effectively, I will do the same after each of the next three treatments as well. These meds are VERY expensive. Bill is calling around for some cost comparisons to see if we can find a better price than the 50 percent co-pay our insurance will cover.

We are in good spirits and optimistic for a full recovery.

Bill worked only two days this past month, between his be-
ing my supporter, bad weather, holidays and appointment
cancellations. He is back to work today. I have tons of
wonderful friends close by to come to my aid and support
as needed, and Katie is just a call away in Port Angeles.
I'm in good hands. I do not think about death, but I don't
think this is denial. It's just that I know this cancer is highly
survivable when caught early and treated aggressively. I
have gotten wonderful information from at least 20 breast
cancer survivors, many of whom say the experience has
made their lives better.

I am working on my memoir about the death of our son,
but that's the closest I come to thinking about death. In re-
membering Scotty's death, and that of my brother, and be-
lieving or knowing that the journey for both the deceased
and the survivor does not have to be negative, I am in no
way depressed by this writing project I've chosen. My writ-
ers group and Alice and nephew Dan have all been very
encouraging and helpful with their suggestions.

This brings us up to date. Keep the warmest thoughts
and prayers coming. I know you are all part of what's mak-
ing this experience acceptable. Love, Cheron 1/20/04

I had 48 good hours during which the anti-nausea medications kept me distress-free. I got lots accomplished at
home and ran a variety of errands in town. On Wednesday
morning that all changed. I awoke with a roaring headache,
vertigo and nausea. Having felt so chipper for the first two
days after treatment, I'd planned to go with a church group
for an outing to a museum followed by lunch in Port Angeles. When the carpool arrived to pick me up at mid-
morning I staggered out to express my regrets, knowing
they'd prefer my absence to seeing me turn green as we
navigated the curvy road to the museum. I loaded up on
meds for nausea and went to bed with Lucy from 10 a.m. to
3 p.m. By then I was much improved so that Lucy and I

could go for a walk to pick up the mail. When we returned we were greeted by my attentive next-door neighbor, Mary, bringing a basket of healthful food. We visited a while, then Lucy and I cuddled in front of the TV to pass the evening in healing mode. Bill had taken to calling Lucy our "mammalian warming blanket" for the comfort her presence brought as she lovingly relaxed beside or on top of one of us.

I had been emailing frequently with Lucy's foster parent, Linda, reporting or asking advice about the dog's adjustment to our home. Feeling much-improved on Thursday, I'd taken Lucy for her vet appointment. I marveled how, coincidentally, Lucy and her eye problem had been cared for, pro bono for the rescue organization, by the vet in <u>our</u> neighborhood and her partner who specialized in animal eye ailments. Linda had driven an hour each way from her home to our county for Lucy's initial cherry-eye surgery. Now I also learned that Dr. Ginny Johnson, one of the two lady vets, was a breast cancer survivor, a second interesting coincidence. After sharing a little about our cancer experiences and scheduling an appointment for Lucy to see Dr. Murphy, the veterinarian eye specialist, I was anxious to email a report of my findings to Linda.

Hi Linda and George: Dr. Johnson saw Lucy this morning and confirms the recurrence of cherry-eye, so we'll take her to see Dr. Murphy on Saturday. Otherwise, Ms. Lucy is doing extraordinarily well after seven weeks in our home. She and Thumb-purr have no intention of sharing our bed amicably yet, but even that relationship continues to get better. I keep the crate in our bedroom and Lucy is fine when I tuck her there for the night…She does well walking with her harness/leash, though still would like to taste a tire when a car goes by on the road. I will give her that kiss you've requested (she is so kissable) and remember you when we enjoy a game of tug-o-war.

I didn't tell you earlier that I was diagnosed with breast cancer the day after Thanksgiving. By the time I met you I'd been through two surgeries to remove the tumor and many lymph nodes under my left arm. By the end of December we were seeing the doctors who are overseeing my continuing treatments, chemo in Bremerton and radiation in Sequim. Bill had been concerned about all the time he's away with his work assignments, and especially wanted me to have a dog for a companion. In truth, I do not feel "unwell" at all, except for several days after extensive surgery, and again yesterday, which was the third day after my first chemo. It was fabulous to have Lucy here with me yesterday when I needed to nap. She stayed right beside me on the pillows for five restful hours. She is a great comfort. Today I feel very good and have already been out for a walk and some errands in town. It's so great that she loves travel in the car because she will go with me to all my appointments. The first four are in Bremerton, and while I'm being infused Bill and Lucy can go for an exercise session at the nearby middle school. When I start daily radiation in Sequim, I can drive myself back and forth. Lucy will be a great asset to keep those trips from becoming tedious. I was somewhat afraid that if I divulged this information about my disease the rescue agency would be reticent to let us adopt Lucy, and that would have been awful! When Bill's away for work, Lucy's the ever-present companion that cares for me.

So, all is going beautifully with Lucy. No regrets, only feelings of gratitude that she's come into our lives. Best regards, Cheron

Linda was quick to reply by email and set my mind at ease:

You don't know me very well but I believe these emails are helping to change that.

If you did, you'd know that I would have protected you and never shared the info about your cancer with the adoption agency if you'd requested me not to do so. It is well-known that dogs have remarkable healing and comforting powers, and I would have gotten Lucy to you much sooner had I known! I pray that the prognosis for you is good and that this nightmare will soon become a distant memory. And, I'm very glad I told you about the harness and even more pleased that you had me pick one up for you. Miss Lucy could have done some serious damage to you if she'd been allowed to pull at her leash. She is so exuberant and strong, I'm amazed she didn't dislocate my shoulder on our walks!

...Dr. Murphy is an excellent surgeon. She did Lucy's surgery the first time. Both of these vet ladies are very loving, very caring, and will take good care of her.

...So much makes sense now – your business in Bremerton on the day I first phoned was a doctor's appointment, right? For certain, Lucy's purpose is to help and comfort you. What a gift and a blessing our dogs are! To think that for a while we considered keeping her when she was destined to be yours all along. Your husband is a very smart man to have wanted a companion for you. If there is ANYTHING I can do, please ask. Linda

I kept daily notes on the Weekly Health Tracker I found in some of the free literature handed out to cancer patients. At the close of week one, I had noted only a half-day when I felt truly awful. Some minor headaches, backaches and intestinal distress were dispelled with various medications and a nap every afternoon. I had returned to my exercise program by pedaling on my stationary bike on Thursday, good preparation for rejoining my aerobics class Friday morning. I recalled the recommendations of Sara, my very first contact after diagnosis, to keep active during the course of treatment.

Friday evening Bill and I attended a potluck supper for church members who were considering traveling with the mission delegation to El Salvador in August. I made a presentation about my prior experiences in our adopted village and encouraged both adults and youth to make the trip. The hostess for the potluck was a nurse who'd already been very supportive, and another whom I was meeting for the first time was eager to share with me about her recent recovery from breast cancer. Nothing at the potluck tasted good because the chemo had caused a metal taste in my mouth. Maybe this was going to be a positive side effect to help allay my fears about gaining excessive weight while being more sedentary than usual.

Saturday morning we received an email from a good friend in Texas divulging that his 33-year-old son had Stage IV melanoma with metastases to his lungs. We were shocked and saddened, but noted the optimism in the message: "Look at Lance Armstrong's recovery and return to amazing strength and good health." I said a prayer for this family and we acknowledged what a comparably better situation we were in.

In contrast to the sadness of this revelation, we were having a good weekend with my treatment regimen finally on schedule and a good prognosis. Bill bathed and brushed Lucy; Katie arrived for a visit during which we teamed up on a trial run of my newly acquired grooming technique. Katie subdued Lucy with sweet talk and caresses, quieting her fear of the noisy electric clippers. Her close-cut head and body felt like velvet while her legs, feet and ears remained curly and fluffy. We removed enough cinnamon-colored hair to stuff a small pillow. The whole process was very rewarding. We agreed that Lucy would be more comfortable and pleasantly fragrant during her upcoming ordeal with eye surgery and post-op confinement.

Monday, one week after the first chemo infusion, I went to the lab in Port Townsend to have my blood drawn, which would become a week-starting ritual for the duration of my chemotherapy. It was necessary to keep careful watch over my red and white cell counts so that I could stave off infection and anemia during the treatment that would predictably lower my resistance and my energy. I noticed that several patients had familiar relationships with the technologists in the lab. I wondered how long they'd been following this blood-check routine, grateful that I didn't have a chronic illness or condition. I was not anticipating this as a lifelong necessity, but one with an end in sight. I was grateful.

A colorful email with many pages of attachments relayed good wishes from a friend by way of quotes attributed to the Dalai Lama and some others. The one that struck me most was by Luciano de Crescenzo: "We are each of us angels with only one wing. And we can only fly embracing each other." How apparently true that was becoming for me as I gratefully acknowledged all of the generous warmth and support I received each and every day.

Dianne hosted dinner for a small group of neighbors. There I met a long-time survivor with whom I compared my situation, realizing again how far we'd advanced in the areas of early diagnosis, treatment, and survivor rates. For the remainder of the week I was symptom-free, able to read and write for hours, making good progress on my manuscript. At midday I took a break for the Tuesday potluck at Dorle's house, where I met a one-year survivor, Sally, who shared the story of her therapy after bilateral mastectomy. As always, I was inspired by Dorle's amazing optimism and courage as she coped with terminal breast cancer that had metastasized to her liver. This remarkable retired teacher and Habitat co-volunteer opened her heart and home, reaching out to a generous group of friends who would share intimately in the final year of her life's journey. I continued to benefit from the growing sisterhood of survivors who kept crossing my path.

Ginger, as always, was a supportive comrade as we worked together in the Habitat re-sale store on Wednesday. Thursday afternoon I enjoyed a visit from a long-time friend, Kim, who had been indispensable in the 1970s when I was completing my dissertation and needed a babysitter for Laura who could communicate in sign language. We'd kept in touch over the years, never suspecting that we'd end up residing in the same town later in life. Kim brought tea and biscotti, as well as Maeve Binche's novel, Quentins, expecting I could use some light reading to fill the hours while recuperating.

Many friends brought or sent books and magazines. Some were sources of knowledge or inspiration for facing crisis, while others provided entertainment or diversion from thinking about cancer. I read The Cancer Conqueror, Waking Samuel, and a book of writings and drawings by the Perskes, inspiring advocates in the field of disability. My Peace Corps buddy, Jamar, sent a lovely book of poetry written to accompany pages of masterpiece paintings by the Dutch artist, Vermeer, whose work was being popularized by a movie titled "Girl with the Pearl Earring." A high school friend, who loved shopping in used bookstores, gathered up a trio of faith inspired books she inscribed with her tender good wishes. College friends in San Diego sent Wit and Wisdom from the Peanut Butter Gang and my youngest sister, Connie, in Florida sent Dog Blessings, both of which brought smiles and chuckles into my days. Sister Alice sent me a subscription to Writers Digest magazine, recognizing my desire to keep the creative juices flowing in order to complete my manuscript. Reading and writing would be important activities during the long days of treatment and healing.

Hats to warm and cover my bald head, as well as snuggly toys, were part of the bounty showered upon me. Our children's godmother, Sue, chose two stylish hats which she sent from Chicago, one of which coordinated perfectly with a favorite hand knit sweater I'd purchased in Ireland years earlier. Christine in Portland, Oregon, a fellow board member with the American Society for Deaf Children, created a matching cloche and muffler of soft, blue, cashmere yarn. A Peace Corps friend in southern California and my son in Missouri each sent a variety of ball caps, one with orange flames and another with stars and stripes adornments. Neighbor Dianne was the first to bring a teddy bear, soft and white, tucked into a hat box decorated by Mary Engelbreit; Alice and Nephew Dan spent a morning at the Build-A-Bear store fashioning a fuzzy purple toy they anointed "Joy" and delivered the weekend before my second chemo treatment; Sister Mary in Spokane chose to support the "race for the cure" by purchasing gifts with the pink-ribbon symbol including a brown, terry-cloth bear, warm socks, and a sticker for the tailgate of my car.

MaryAnna in Texas, a friend whose breast cancer would be diagnosed six months later, chose for me a pewter bracelet inscribed: "Guardian Angel, Protect and Guide; be always at my side." Because of Lance Armstrong's success in launching an international fundraiser and cancer awareness campaign which marketed yellow rubber, "Livestrong" bracelets, these were provided by several friends. I also received similar ones in bright pink and baby blue to support the same activities on behalf of breast cancer and prostate cancer. I wore them all at the same time, every day and night, even in the shower. Mickey, a professor friend in Oregon, supplied fragrant lotion and bath salts to pamper my skin and soothe my spirits.

My hair still seemed firmly rooted and I felt "all together" when I headed for Seattle on January 30, nearly two full weeks after the start of chemotherapy. After visiting my mother and the other residents at her assisted living home, I drove another hour for the semi-annual gathering of my Franklin High School "gal pals" group. The six of us ate a wholesome lunch and laughed heartily as we remembered old times and reviewed some of our experiences during the intervening 48 years of our post-high school lives. Each friend had an offering of support: Gail would send me copies of school newspapers from 1960 as reference material for my memoir; Linda was eager to provide books with inspiring messages; Diane made herself available to edit my manuscript when I was ready. Wendy, whose breast cancer treatment had been completed only months earlier, shared her wisdom and advice. I learned from her about the differential diagnosis among breast cancer patients, whose tumors were determined to be either "receptor negative" or "receptor positive," and the effect this had on the course of treatment. If estrogen had facilitated the cancer growth, as in my case, the patient would benefit from a long-term estrogen-blocking medication. Whereas Wendy, being estrogen negative, was taking no follow-up drugs. I'd been told I would have a daily dose of Tamoxifen or similar medication prescribed for at least five years after completing radiation.

Who needs hair, anyway!?

On February 2, my hair began clogging the shower drain. Only six days later I looked a lot like Sigorney Weaver in the movie, "Alien." When Daughter Katie came for her weekend visit she was easily persuaded to finish the job by giving me a buzz cut using Lucy's dog grooming clippers. Hair loss was the major symptom I noted in my weekly health tracker booklet, but I was also experiencing some insomnia, backache, toothache, scalp itch and genital irritation. I had pills to address each of these maladies. Bill joked, "Better living through chemistry." I gratefully embraced the magic potions concocted by those wizards of science! Generally, I took meds very cautiously and sparingly, but the doctors now in my life encouraged me to address my discomfort aggressively, before it became unmanageable. So, I popped pills, and they did wonders to restore my sense of wellbeing.

Baldness became the most striking change in my behavior or appearance, but it was fun donning the myriad hats and wigs I had gathered in my arsenal. I wore a "topper" 24/7, including the nighttime turbans loaned to me from the cosmetology project at the trade school. The first Sunday "AB" – After Balding – I chose to wear golden, shoulder-length tresses with full bangs. My support entourage – Sister Alice, Daughter Katie, and Niece Dayna – sat with me near the back of the sanctuary. I realized a sense of anonymity, as if I were disguised or visiting incognito. I felt like an impish tease as familiar people looked quizzical or embarrassed, then looked away, confused by the inability to identify this vaguely familiar visage in their midst. Geri, from her spot in the distant choir loft, studied my face with a curious frown for several gazes before breaking into a broad grin upon recognition of her neighbor who'd been transformed from a middle-aged brunette into a blonde bombshell.

I found myself analyzing the ebb and flow of my cancer-directed life from my perspective as a professional counselor, and from my memories of confronting various adversities during my lifetime.

"The human organism seeks equilibrium" – a basic truism learned in my college sociology and psychology courses, and observable in my life passage. This unbidden and unwelcome disease has thrown a monkey wrench into my plans for my life approaching the "golden years," yet the ongoing days and weeks don't seem horribly upsetting or unmanageable. With confidence in God's plan for me, and the support of family and friends, I anticipate full recovery and find plenty of calm enjoyment every single day. I'm remembering my work with families raising kids with

disabilities, and how the literature often talked about help-
ing them survive their challenges and burdens. Seems to me
that survival is too basic a goal, at least for most of us in
Western societies where so much more is attainable. I ex-
pect to THRIVE again, probably stronger for having con-
fronted this disease with refusal to let it conquer my spirit.
The goal should be "thrivival" rather than survival. My
mind/body-self fights for balance everyday, and then my
spirit-self takes over to go the extra mile toward thrivival –
hope, joy, and positive expectations for the future.

The prayer chain at First Presbyterian Church started
sending supplications on my behalf as soon as I revealed
my diagnosis. More prayers came from folks I didn't even
know in my daughter-in-law's Lutheran church in southeast
Missouri, and a former coworker in Eugene, Oregon asked
his Episcopal congregation to pray for my healing. I figured
this ecumenical outpouring of prayer buoyed my chances of
a good outcome. I was conscious of being encircled by a
boundless loving energy. I basked in the warmth of it,
grateful for the tender mercies streaming toward me from
all sides.

Compassion inspires true friends to surmount obstacles
in order to be there for you. Many people traveled long dis-
tances to spend time with me. Their helpful visits were
priceless gifts to energize me through those seven months
of treatment. Julie and Peter drove from northeastern Oregon as soon as the winter weather permitted. Seeing Lucy's
restlessness in confinement, they mapped a course for a
long walk through the woods and along the beachfront. It
wouldn't have been a wise venture on my own, but with
them it was a chance to test my endurance, getting a
healthy dose of fresh air while Lucy experienced the joy of
romping and sniffing all along the way.

My nephew, David, brought his newborn son from Seattle for a Valentine visit. Settled in my easy chair, I soaked

up the sight, sound and smells of this tiny bundle in my arms. Lucy waited at my feet with patience and curiosity when she wasn't playing tug-o-war with Baby Dawson's proud sister, Dayna. Having the two children nearby helped ameliorate the longing for my only grandson, a toddler living 2,000 miles away in Missouri. My sister, Mary, and her husband, Keith, drove from western Washington, bearing gifts to cheer me.

On February 5th I picked up Dorle, who'd invited me to a breast cancer support group at the local hospital. We were the only two patients who showed up. Because I'd facilitated many self-help groups over the years, and because Dorle was a seasoned and well-informed patient, the session seemed superfluous for the two of us, though we were able to help the young woman who was learning to lead the group! Dorle and I had already shared most of our thoughts and feelings about the cancer journey, but we were willing to review all this to educate the facilitator-in-training. I went to this monthly session only once again, later in the spring, when an older woman called asking me to drive her there. The group was now a triad – Dorle, this new woman and me – but the three of us were happy to spend the hour chatting and sharing while yet another young medical social worker used the time to listen and observe.

I was feeling almost normal in the week prior to my second chemo treatment. I had energy to attend meetings, visit with friends, prepare and mail Valentine gift boxes for my children, and work on my memoir several hours most days. Because my blood test results showed a low white blood count of 1.3, I called the nurse in Bremerton to see if it would affect my treatment schedule. She explained that this dip was to be expected a week into the three-week chemo cycle, and that my WBC was likely now on the rise in the days preparatory to another infusion. She warned me to stay away from sick people and potential infections, but otherwise stay as active as energy allowed.

The storyline in my memoir-novel had reached a place where I was imagining and creating a chapter in which my son, Scotty, was cementing relationships with new friends in his heavenly home. I attributed to Divine Inspiration my decision to pair the true story of our recovery after Scotty's death with a parallel, "novel" tale about his new life in Heaven. Writing these imaginary passages gave me respite from the sorrow of recounting our course through grief work, and I believed my readers would similarly benefit from this writing convention. I'd interviewed Ginger for details about the appearance and personality of her four-year-old, Steve, who'd died at nearly the same age only a few years before the car accident that took Scotty's life in 1977. Creating a roommate relationship and scenario for the little boys in Heaven was a delightful exercise for me, even while I grieved again for my child as I looked at picture albums and handled the precious belongings we'd saved to remind us of his short life in our family.

Alice brought her granddaughter, Dayna, from Seattle for our pre-treatment weekend of fun. Katie and her greyhound, Lexi, joined us on Saturday for a beach picnic preceding a visit to the earthquake exhibit at the Marine Science Center. Sunday we all went to church and a Sunday matinee at Port Townsend's vintage Rose Theater for a benefit showing of "Calendar Girls," a comical movie about middle-aged women defying social conventions in England. It was a beautiful winter weekend with no wind or rain, and some sun breaks. My golden tresses sparkled, camouflaging my baldness. My hairdo was similar to the styles worn by both Dayna and Katie, so we appeared as three generations of blonde bombshells!

The second chemo infusion went off without a hitch. The nurse had little trouble finding a good vein, and my secret sister from church, Mary Ann, came by to visit with me. The three-hour process passed quickly. Mary Ann was the neighbor friend who had "secretly" sent her husband dressed as Santa Claus to present me with a poinsettia the week before Christmas, when I was recovering from the lumpectomy. Later she would be one of my drivers for radiation treatments in Sequim. In July she graciously offered her home for overflow lodging of wedding guests, as well as lending a hand with all the floral arrangements. She was a wonderful extra sister!

With Lucy's eye surgery scheduled for February 11, I was glad this week after chemo was easy. I felt a bit "druggy" and needed medication for a nagging backache, but not too fatigued to run errands, attend meetings and even exercise a little on the elliptical trainer at home. Doggie surgery and follow-up appointments went well, and neighbor Mary prepared a Valentine dinner for Bill and me on Saturday.

I composed my email Update to a group of 44 friends and relatives, "Two chemo zaps down, two to go!" I preceded the message with a photo of Alice and four gorgeous blondes – Katie, Dayna, Thumb-purr and me – taken after our movie outing the prior weekend.

My second chemo was easier than the first. Only one stick to find a good vein. A visit while I was being infused from one of my favorite neighbors. Lucy comes along to keep Bill company on the trips to Bremerton, and the two of them enjoy "doggie-master quality time" walking on the track at a nearby school until I'm ready to be chauffeured back home.

My oncologist said I tolerated the first three-week treatment regimen very well and shouldn't expect it to get any worse. I have my last treatment on March 22 and should be recovered and ready for radiation any time after April 12. So, I'm feeling pretty good.

I am bald. A couple of my supporters have told me I have a lovely shaped head! But I've decided not to scare anyone with the bare facts. Instead I'm having fun with many different caps, hats and wigs. At least a dozen of you have provided me with "toppers" for my head. Others have kept the cards, books, gifts, supportive keepsakes, phone calls and emails coming. Locals have brought food or cooked meals. Sincere thanks to all. You are precious to me and vital to my recovery.

We have friends on this cancer journey who are having a much harder time than I am, so I don't mean to be flippant or Pollyanna about the whole thing. I certainly do need all your prayers and support, but I do NOT need you to worry, okay? Bill and I are starting to plan a summer trip to Europe in celebration of my return to good health. We think the future is bright. Love, Cheron

I was a bit taken back when our friend Richard, in Austin, replied to this Update, which I'd attached to an email on a different subject. He wrote, "I didn't ask about your health situation." Pondering his words made me realize I needed to be more sensitive to the recipients chosen for my newsy reports. Richard and his wife, Liz, were struggling in the aftermath of learning about their young adult son's more serious cancer, and feeling overwhelmed with the challenges his treatment imposed. I needed to discern which of the folks on my list were going to appreciate four months of my self-disclosure, and which were going to find it overkill. My intention was to be informative about the disease as well as my progress through treatment. Perhaps it would be wise to limit the Updates, at least after successful completion of chemotherapy.

Lucy's "cherry-eye" problem was resolved with surgery on February 11. Caring for her post-op was a joy, returning the favor for all the comfort she had showered on me with her loving presence during this cancer ordeal. She had patiently allowed me on-the-job training as a groomer, which was most rewarding. As her eyes became clear, she was a real cinnamon beauty with the sweet personality to match her appearance.

The persistent backache defied my use of pain medication, which challenged my determination to keep up a normal pace of life through the remainder of February. I went to church and a number of meetings where I could sit and participate only nominally, but trying to work my half-day shift at the Habitat store wore me out. I napped more and experimented with more medication for migraines and stomachaches, which likely were exacerbated by the medication for backache! I slept and lay around much more than usual, my body finally responding positively as the next chemo appointment approached.

During this down time I started planning in earnest for upcoming travels that we had deemphasized while needing to focus on the present-day demands of treatment and recovery. Alice had sent me an email back in January with the essential message, "Don't cancel life!" I had gone ahead with Katie's graduation party while still recovering from two surgeries and wearing the ugly drain tube under my dress-up clothes, and the shortened trip to Palm Springs lifted my spirits as I approached the initiation of chemotherapy in January. Now I looked forward to surprising my fellow board member when our national meeting was to be held in Portland during early March, wearing my best blonde wig! I made lodging reservations for four of us along the route of Missouri's Katy Trail, which we planned to navigate by bicycle in April, anxious also to see our grandson in St. Louis while in the Midwest. The 40th reunion of my college class would occur in June. In late-July we'd scheduled the river cruise from Basel, Switzerland to Amsterdam, with hopes of riding bikes in the low countries of Belgium and Holland before returning to the U.S. This was the graduation gift we'd promised Katie. Indeed, I was determined not to "cancel life" and miss out on these adventures and reunions with loved ones.

On March 28 Alice and her son, Daniel, arrived for our pre-chemo gathering intent on preparing a gourmet meal together. After church we shared abundant laughter around the kitchen counters while creating a tasty feast for our leap-day lunch on Sunday. Katie and her beau, Ryan, joined us for chicken cordon bleu and a decadent frozen yogurt dessert, followed by three rounds of Scrabble. After they left for Seattle and Port Angeles, Julie called from eastern Oregon to report on her plans to be in Port Townsend after April 19. Julie, being one of my closest, long-standing soul mates, spoke words of encouragement in warm and wonderful tones. She always put me in touch with my spiritual core, so that I found myself meditating in that sphere after her call.

The fruit of the spirit

"...the fruit of the Spirit is love, joy, peace...patience, kindness, goodness, faithfulness, gentleness, self-control..."
These Biblical words, commonly found on wall hangings and bookmarks, had a calming effect as I grappled with the need for greater patience. Again and again this cancer journey was forcing me to accept delay and disappointment with grace. I was forced to relinquish control in some aspects of my life, but still believed the tenet I'd learned in childhood, "God helps those who help themselves." It occurred to me that this was the great test of life: How to strike a peaceable balance between self-control and giving over to the will of God. How to relax and let life take its course, but to continue striving and doing whatever possible to improve a troublesome situation. Rev. Slater had preached a sermon based on one of Jesus' parables, calling for us to avoid the neurotic negativism that made us dissatisfied with our situations. I was determined to maintain a positive mindset, confident that I would be healthier and happier for doing so.

Following the third infusion session in Bremerton on Monday morning, the first of March, I experienced the usual sense of wellness and energy. I took a dessert I'd prepared and enjoyed the camaraderie of the lunch crowd at Dorle's house. On Wednesday morning I worked my shift at the Habitat store but was feeling peaked by noon, whereupon I drove home for a nap. It took me the rest of the week to stabilize and overcome the inertia and malaise. When I composed my email Update on March 7, I chose to start off with a photo of Bill and me relaxing and smiling, holding Lucy and Thumb-purr in our laps.

I chose this picture to go with the quote I recently read, "Individuals don't get cancer, families do." This is our everyday family of four, including the two pets. I earlier reported to some of you that Lucy was having a difficult time respecting the cat and there was a lot of chasing and barking going on. This picture is to demonstrate that we are getting closer to a peaceable kingdom around here. Thumb-purr has realized he needs to assert himself as the <u>lion</u> to reduce Lucy to the <u>lamb</u>. Though Lucy still wants the cat to engage in puppy play, they are quite tolerant of each other. They both like the privilege of sleeping on our bed, and almost kiss in the morning. It has been a great comfort to have a furry friend on each side of me when I'm down and feeling crummy.

I have felt crummier this go-round. My third chemo treatment was a week ago and it's taken all these days to stabilize enough to compose an Update. The cumulative effects of the chemicals have caught up with me and I've experienced more symptoms than in the early going. I have a metal taste in my mouth all the time (brush teeth frequently and suck on peppermints). There are stomach pains and some dehydration. Now the chemicals are doing their job of killing off fast-growing cells all through my body, but that includes red blood cells, so I'm anemic. I've started taking

90

exorbitantly expensive shots of erythropoietin (Epo, Pro-crit) to get cell production going again. Bill took on the task of comparison shopping with pharmacies and negoti-ating with our insurance company, again. I'll get these weekly shots for five weeks until I'm well past the last infu-sion on March 22. Should help with the fatigue and my need for naps most days.

So, I am now at seven weeks down and five to go, with just one infusion remaining. In between the end of chemo and the start of daily radiation treatments, we are going on a trip to Missouri to see grandson Jeremy and to bike on the famous Katy Trail with our cycling friends from Salem, Noel and Myrna. Radiations will take up most of May and June.

I've gotten way behind with my housework and will probably invite my friend Ginger to vacuum while I dust next week. I tried to do a little on Friday, but only suc-ceeded in spilling a puddle of blue Windex all over the tan carpet. Decided I was too "frail" to be doing housework! Don't really miss it, and both Bill and I are getting accus-tomed to a bit more dirt than usual. Not a high priority.

I don't like losing a whole week's work on my writing with every infusion, but I just don't have a creative brain when my body is handling the chemicals. I have also been distressed with the news that one of my closest college gal pals, with whom I sang in a quintet, died of cancer on Feb-ruary 13. We are vulnerable and not invincible, no matter how strong we seek to keep our spirits. All we can do is take each day as it comes with hope and courage. I know, or suspect, that some of you are experiencing challenges that require this sort of effort as well. You are in my prayers and I feel oneness with you in your suffering.

There are many ways in which I know I am lucky, be-yond all this "family" I have pulling for me. I am lucky to have been inspired and enabled by Bill to get a grip on my health care twelve years ago so that I lost 100 pounds and arned the importance of daily exercise. I'm positive I'd be less able to manage this cancer if I were at a miserable 236 pounds! I'm lucky because I was able to retire at age 55 to devote my energies to volunteer work that I love, and to enjoy a less stressful lifestyle. We are lucky that we can handle the costs of cancer care. I know that many people die because they don't have the resources to face this disease aggressively.

We continue to be upbeat most of the time. Thanks again for your continued prayers and comforting thoughts. Love, Cheron (and Bill)

On March 11th I gratefully accepted Ginger's offer to help me with housework. The place had been generally neglected since she came to vacuum and assist with preparations for Katie's graduation party in December. There was a layer of dust on most surfaces, dust bunnies in corners and under furniture, and cobwebs higher up that were beginning to show as spring sunshine frequently beamed through our windows. The next morning I wrote a thank you note to Ginger:

It's 7:30 and I'm just getting the pets fed and starting the day. I took a sleeping pill last night because my sleep has been irregular lately, and it worked. A good night's rest, for a change.

When I came out to the kitchen, I was impressed with my feeling of wellbeing. It's raining at the moment, so I'm not being uplifted by the sunshine and vistas. I realize that my contentment is in looking around the house and seeing it CLEAN! That's right: I'm thrilled to enjoy the cleanliness after it had gotten way ahead of me for several weeks. A clean and orderly house makes me feel so good.

It has reminded me of the experience after Scotty was killed, people bringing scads of food to our family. It all started happening so quickly and there was SO MUCH of *it! The refrigerator and freezer soon became filled to ca-pacity, even as our appetites were dulled and eating seemed so unimportant. The whole idea of people bringing food and more food seemed so old-fashioned to me, and I was inclined to reject it if anyone asked in advance before just showing up with a meal.*

But I came to realize that food-offerings are one of the very tangible and practical ways that friends can be most helpful in times of grief and agony. If it hadn't been for all that food, we probably wouldn't have been very well nour-ished during that first month or two. And I would have been challenged to be a good hostess to people who came by to visit with us. As it was, I had treats that I could serve with coffee or tea, and something for any children who wanted to see our surviving son, Phillip. The most important thing was that I would have been a wreck if I'd had to spend much time in the grocery store, for food shopping had be-come a favorite play and learning time for me with the boys. I'll write about that in my memoir.

So, Ginger, I just wanted to let you know that your idea of helping with housework is MOST EXCELLENT! I'm not a total invalid and probably could be keeping up much bet-ter than I am, but I'm sure not inspired to do so day by day. Saving my energy for things that are more necessary and more enjoyable seems okay...I can allow myself to do it. But, eventually the rugs really DO need to be vacuumed well and all that dust and pet hair cleaned up!

You are a jewel of a friend, perceptive and caring to a fault. I just wanted you to know all this as I'm observing my own reaction to a CLEAN HOUSE this morning. It perks up and frees my spirit. I thank God for your friendship. Love, Cheron

Katie and Alice joined 30 church friends and me on March 13 at a forested convention site where we celebrated the annual Presbyterian Women's Retreat. Mary Brunner was very attentive, welcoming and loving the three of us as if we were her biological family.

The overnight get away was refreshing and fun. The Epo injections were working to "pump me up," an expression Bill borrowed from the Hans and Franz characters of the Saturday Night Live cast. During early March I felt well enough to attend the full schedule of meetings and events penciled on my calendar: Dorle's Tuesday lunch potlucks, shifts at the Habitat store, vet appointments with Lucy, Trustees meeting and Grief Recovery group at church, my writers' group, AAUW meeting, dinner parties hosted by neighbors Mary, Dianne and the Lowes, and a Habitat committee work session.

On March 20 my pre-chemo gang arrived from Seattle to cheer me on. Katie, Alice, her son and her two granddaughters, took me out for dinner at Ajax Café where we donned crazy hats and laughed a lot.

Erythropoietin is a magic potion! Considering it's positive effects with me, it is almost understandable that riders competing in the Tour de France might try to get some into their systems! Just two days after my final chemo treatment, I sent this Update:

Hi everyone: I'm pleased to report that my last chemo session occurred in Bremerton on Monday, and it went smoothly. I left the clinic with congrats from my oncology nurse and a sense of great relief for both Bill and me. My first-day symptom was double vision, but now I'm back to "metallic mouth" with some wooziness. When we got home Monday afternoon, Bill fired up the lawnmower to cut the long damp grass for the first time since fall. I got out my rake and broom to help with clean up, but he swiftly dispatched me back indoors to less rigorous pursuits or rest. "You've just had a half-gallon of toxic chemicals run into your body and there's no need to be doing yard work!" So, the lawn looks pretty good, but the weeds will continue to thrive in all the flower beds until I'm back to the rigors of gardening.

The Procrit injections have brought my red blood cell count up to an acceptable 35, and my white count is satisfactory. I'm grateful that I have not had any overlay of bacterial or viral infections during this time of lowered resistance. Evidently many people get mouth sores, skin problems, bad colds, etc. I have not had to contend with any of that.

This three-week cycle will end April 11, at which time the toxins should have cleared my body and I'll start feeling more normal. Hair re-growth is not expected to be significant until summertime. There will be break time before the start of daily radiation treatments in Sequim on May 3. That's not supposed to be anywhere near as difficult, just tiring and some possible burning of the breast tissue. After radiation I'll probably be on oral Tamoxifen for five years, then another oral hormone treatment for an additional five years. My oncologist seems to think I have at least ten good treatment years ahead of me.

We have a trip to Missouri planned, beginning April 23. First we'll visit with our grandson and his family in St. Louis, then we'll meet our Salem cycling friends to bike the Katy Trail, west to east, across the whole of Missouri. Bill assured Dr. Murphy that we'd be able to catch a train and curtail the trip if I find I can't manage it, but she didn't seem to be worried about it. The course is pretty flat and we will stay in B&Bs or hotels so we can sleep decent nights between legs on the trail. We'll end in St. Charles, near St. Louis, then fly to San Diego for a two-day orthopedics meeting on May 1-2.

I have finished writing about one-third of my novel-memoir and sent it off yesterday to two friends with professional credentials, one an editor/journalist, and one a publisher. I'm hoping they can give me some good advice as I continue this creative journey. If I don't encounter unfore-

seen problems or challenges, it's possible I will complete the first draft by year's end.

We continue to be deeply grateful for all the support I receive every day from you, my cyber buddies. I'll try to get a good picture of our Katy Trail adventure for my next Update. Until then, thanks a million. Love, Cheron

Darlene Toole, my deaf friend who is both an author and breast cancer survivor, had invited Bill and me to stay at her house when we went to Portland for the meeting of the ASDC Board. The three friends who knew I was hoping to join the group for dinner had kept the secret so that my entrance to the restaurant was a joyous, welcoming surprise for the rest. These twelve people, with whom I shared a deep commitment to the welfare of kids with hearing loss, had become good friends though we only met face to face once or twice a year. Email communication kept us connected so that all were aware of my cancer. But, they didn't expect to see me in my blonde bombshell wig surrounding a healthy, happy, smiling face. It proved to be a wonderful reunion, made even better because Darlene and I had time to spend comparing progress and encouraging each other toward good health.

With less than a month to prepare for the long bike trip across Missouri, I had to get in the saddle for serious training. Bill made a trailer in which he could pull Lucy behind his bike. The three of us set out for an excellent trail emanating from Carrie Blake Park in Sequim. We intended to ride five to ten miles for my first outing, then increase the distance by ten miles each of the ensuing weeks. That way I'd be ready to ride at least 40 miles each day of the trip. Five miles, with a little uphill, turned out to be too great a challenge so soon after chemo. I lagged behind Bill and Lucy after two miles, then wobbled to a halt at about mile three, afraid I was going to faint with exhaustion! Back home for a shot of that magic, pump-up potion, Erythropoietin, and two days later I was more than capable of pedaling ten miles. The next week I went 20, then 30, and could easily have managed 40 by the last week of my training regimen.

Spring into action

Before we flew off to St. Louis, we delighted in a visit from my sister and her husband from Spokane, Mary and Keith. We took the ferry out of Pt. Townsend to hike across Ft. Casey on Whidbey Island. The fresh sea air was invigorating, as was the hike. It was only two days later when Julie and Peter arrived from LaGrande, OR. They, too, helped me test my increasing endurance as we hiked the wooded trails and sandy beaches near our home with Lucy happily in tow.

In mid-April, Katie sent a brief email message announcing that Ryan had asked her to marry him! Since I'd had a couple similar proposals I'd agreed to before meeting Bill – both of which dreams dissolved within months – I was only moderately excited. Bill queried, "Did she say 'Yes'?" and remarked that Ryan hadn't approached him for his permission! During the ensuing week, Katie confirmed her intention to marry her young Coast Guard beau, and Ryan wrote a heartfelt note that constituted his request for Katie's hand in marriage. When the two sat down with me at the dining room table to discuss their desire to be married in July, I suggested they might try a longer engagement with more time to discuss and plan for their lifetime together. However, they were looking ahead to early fall when Ryan would be transferred for a training program in Virginia, then to another duty station after that. They were intent on sharing these new adventures as husband and wife. We determined that July 10 was best in everyone's schedule, and then set about making detailed arrangements for a major celebration that had to come together in less than three months. This diversion was a godsend to keep me happily occupied throughout radiation treatments, and to anticipate as a thrilling conclusion after my long months of aggressive cancer care.

We'd been planning the 200-mile bike trip since fall and before my diagnosis, so it was fortuitous that the dates coincided with the month-long break between chemo and radiation. I never considered canceling this outing because it provided a goal, which inspired my exercise program as I worked to keep my body strong, and kept my spirits up as I looked forward to fun and recreation in America's heartland. The west-to-east course we'd plotted started south of Kansas City, following part of the route taken by Lewis and Clark 200 years earlier, and ending in St. Charles, near St. Louis. The course was part of the rails-to-trails conversion of old train tracks into hiking and biking paths that was occurring all across the nation. There would be no steep and formidable upgrades. We had reserved comfortable lodging in interesting locations about every 40 miles along the way.

Thankfully, my body seemed recovered from chemotherapy treatments and responsive to the training in which Bill and I had engaged during the preparatory month. I was able to easily manage the miles of pedaling, and we enjoyed the camaraderie of Noel and Myrna, with whom we had made two similar trips to the San Juan Islands and the Gulf Islands in Canada. At the midway point in Jefferson City, I had arranged to visit over dinner with my good friend, Natalie, who had succeeded me as president of the American Society for Deaf Children. Her family lived in the vicinity. Natalie also had a co-worker who was just beginning her chemotherapy for breast cancer. The morning after our dinner together, Myrna and I were quite content to tarry a while with Natalie and Becky while Bill and Noel forged onward along the Katy Trail. After a ladies' leisurely morning, the four of us went in Natalie's SUV to meet the guys 40 miles further east, then commenced the remainder of that day's leg along the trail to our bed-and-breakfast destination for the evening.

We packed our bicycles to return to Port Townsend via UPS, and then Bill and I flew from St. Louis to San Diego for his orthopedics conference. For me it was an opportunity to spend a couple days with longtime friends, Dale and Kendra Dawson. Dale had been a classmate at Pacific University 40 years earlier and we'd remained close over the decades, both spending careers in the people-helping professions. The Dawsons invited us for dinner and took me to the famed San Diego Zoo during the day while Bill was busy. I was comfortable with my baldness covered with just a baseball cap, cooler in the San Diego sun than if I'd worn a wig. On May 3 we flew back to Washington to begin my radiation treatments.

Update, 5/5/04: Hi All: We arrived back Sunday night from our trip to Missouri. It featured a nice visit with our darling grandson, Jeremy, then execution of the long-planned bike ride on the famous rails-to-trails, Katy Trail. I'm pleased to report that we biked west to east in 4.5 days, Bill riding 225 miles and I, 185 miles. The surface was more difficult than we anticipated, so the going was slow and required perseverance, but all four of us (including our Salem biking buddies, Noel and Myrna) completed the challenge. I feel very affirmed in that I'm regaining strength and stamina post-chemo. No hair, but strong heart, lungs and muscles!

After three mid-April radiation prep days during which doctors and techs poked me, drew diagrams and tattoos on my breasts, and ran me through all sorts of big medical devices, I had my first zap yesterday. It's a piece of cake. I'll have these easy treatments daily for 33 total, which will take me through mid-June. I suspect the hardest part will be all the commuting to the oncology center that is 30 miles away in Sequim. Many of my girlfriends here are going to chauffeur me about half of the days, which will make the outings more positive. The possible side effects are fatigue and some burning of the breast tissue, but I'm not taking any time to worry about that at this juncture...

...because I have more important things to occupy my time and energy. Katie decided in mid-April to marry her Coast Guard beau, Ryan Wyman, on July 10. His family is from Valencia, CA. We are in a whirl of wedding planning. The ceremony will be here in our historic Presbyterian Church, and the reception in the Bishop Victorian Gardens. I'm learning and re-learning all sorts of event planning skills, and meeting new folks all over town. This lovely Victorian seaport is actually a fantastic place to hold a wedding with so many excellent providers to help you spend down your wedding budget! In addition, we have a whole passel of local friends, neighbors and relatives who are donating their wonderful skills, time and energy. I couldn't manage without them.

I don't have access right now to any photos of us biking, but I'll attach an engagement picture of the happy couple. Please continue to keep us in your thoughts and prayers, both in regard to the cancer challenges and our activities as parents of the bride. Love, Cheron

Neighbor Dianne took the list I'd been making of all the women who'd asked to be called "if there was anything at all" they could do to help. Her phone calls and coordination efforts set up a schedule so that I had fourteen friends driving me to and from the sessions in Sequim approximately every other treatment day. These were occasions for me to get better acquainted with this supportive group of ladies, often extending our time together by having lunch at a restaurant along the way. The waiting room at the radiation oncology center had an awe-inspiring view of the snow-capped Olympic Mountains, and there was always a jigsaw puzzle in progress on the corner table. I love jigsaw puzzles and found that Geri, my neighbor and friend from church, also harbored a passion for the interlocking pieces. The day she drove we got engaged in the puzzle for a few minutes until I was called. When I returned to the waiting room ten minutes later I sat down and we continued puzzling for a long time, thoroughly enjoying ourselves and oblivious to the time. When we finally communicated about the trip back home, I realized that Geri thought I was still waiting for treatment. I told her I'd finished 45 minutes earlier, but didn't want to disturb her puzzle progress, preferring to seat myself and join the fun!

The first 30 radiation treatments were carefully focused on an area about eight inches square that had been mapped under the direction of the oncologist. To create this "field," the techs had applied three, small, purple tattoos for demarcation. I had to laugh as I recalled all the times Bill and I had indicated to our children our distaste for tattooing, which had come into vogue as body art. Now I was joining the three of them who had defied our wishes! However, I mused, mine would never be visible to anyone short of my husband and medical caretakers. The final three treatments of the 33 would be much more targeted to the immediate area from which the tumor had been removed. I learned later that this regimen is carefully tailored to the patient. For example, some of the women I talked with had tumors already larger than 2cc when diagnosed, and that often meant they could benefit by having the tumor radiated first in hopes it could be shrunken and the surgery would be less pervasive.

May flew by quickly with all the planning for the wedding, as well as my dedication to writing my memoir-novel. Midday trips and treatments simply created a break in days filled with other activities, mostly enjoyable since I was feeling so healthy and confident with light at the end of the treatment tunnel. Katie was searching for a gown when she had time off from substitute teaching in Port Angeles. I wasn't invited to join her on the shopping excursions. Instead, I was coming to terms with the fact that my daughter would never be wearing the velveteen, fur-trimmed gown I'd worn in my winter wedding nearly 38 years earlier. I'd had it professionally cleaned and hermetically sealed. We'd hauled and stored it as we moved around the country during our marriage. But Katie would need a summer-weight dress, to say nothing of her obvious preference for a modern, more revealing gown. She did a good job finding one that was reasonably priced, being as dedicated as I was to staying within a budget and not getting victimized or price-gouged during this vulnerable time. I was happy to be able to coordinate a whole host of other plans and processes for the big event.

The determination for a July wedding also accommodated the previous plans we'd made to take Katie to Europe as a graduation gift in August. When, in April, the couple came to discuss their hopes about marriage, part of the conversation centered on the convenience of having a potential "honeymoon" already in the works. They suggested that Ryan might buy his ticket to join the three of us on a European river cruise and bike trip in Holland, making a very special honeymoon more monetarily feasible. We all laughed at the prospect of the parents going along on what was supposed to be a very intimate get-away for the newlyweds, but both Ryan and Katie thought it was a fine idea. So this became one more phase of the planning for a wonderful summer, having lots of relaxed time to become better acquainted with our delightful new son.

A negative occurrence during this period was the development and exacerbation of lymphedema, or swelling, in my left arm and side. Though not evident to the casual observer, I was aggravated by the tingling, sometimes painful sensation of fullness around the surgical site. The surgeon had removed 21 lymph nodes during lumpectomy, even though none showed any sign of cancer metastasis.

From the literature and reports of other breast cancer survivors, I'd learned that the usual procedure was to biopsy the sentinel node during the operation, and then proceed according to the evidence of cancer spread or containment. My friend, Sara, had had several nodes removed until they found a few that were cancer free and were confident that they'd curtailed the spread in her lymphatic system. To this day it seems excessive that so many of my non-cancerous nodes had been removed, leaving my left arm and side compromised and aggravated. I was sent for therapy to increase range of motion and strengthen the arm, and I was fitted with a compression sleeve. The improvement was negligible. The situation has remained during the ensuing years, somewhat restricting the use of my left arm and causing discomfort when I try to sleep on that side. I was told this condition was also worsened by radiation.

There was also the "Cancer Support Diet." Because cancer is an "obligate glucose feeder," it needs sugar and other carbohydrates to live and grow. A diet high in fiber, low in fat, and as organic as possible was suggested. All forms of sugar were to be avoided.

This is not a lot different from weight-reduction diets I have been aware of and pursuing most of my life. As if tendency toward overweight wasn't bad enough, now I have a life-and-death threat pushing me to forego my favorite foods, most of which would be considered desserts. What a bummer. Cancer doesn't give one much leeway for vices, not even eating!

Lots of vegetables, except corn; moderate amounts of fresh fruits and juices; whole grains, legumes, soy nuts and seeds; mushrooms and "limited free-range poultry"; salmon, mackerel, herring and sardines; avoidance of dairy, fried and microwaved foods and all the dangerous saturated fats and their sources, like beef and lamb. I convinced myself to try these restrictions, but not to impose them rigidly. I wasn't willing to become an absolute slave to this disease, which I truly believed was being cured by surgery, chemotherapy and radiation.

In late June we went to Pacific University's alumni weekend to celebrate my class's 40th reunion. I was as slim as I'd been in years, my blonde-bombshell wig made me look more youthful than my brown locks had looked in years, and I was riding high in my attitude of gratitude for being alive to share this day with my college friends.

Wedding plans progressed and everything fell into place beautifully. Katie and Ryan took charge of several aspects, consulting me for ideas and checking to see what fit our budget. Ryan's parents were wonderful and anxious to help in any way. Mary, my next door neighbor, wanted to provide fancy sandwiches as the mainstay of the mid-afternoon garden reception. She planned to gather the ingredients and a work party to prepare the finger food the morning of the wedding. I wanted to do all the flowers ourselves, enlisting a talented group of six friends to create corsages, bouquets, boutonnières, flower crowns for the candle lighters and table centerpieces, the day before the ceremony. A neighbor who lived down the block, but whom I'd seldom seen, had come by in May to offer vases she'd used for her niece's wedding. She told me she'd just completed her radiation treatments at the same facility where mine were underway, and she knew the competent staff there very well. Amazingly, the "sisterhood" of survivors was continuing to grow all around me!

From x-ray to the altar

On May 28th I celebrated my final radiation treatment with a seafood lunch in a popular Sequim restaurant, hosted by my longtime friend from college, Anne, who had retired on the Peninsula. Afterwards we drove around the area to visit the lavender farms for which Sequim has become famous. Now all that remained on the therapy schedule was a visit with my oncologist to determine the oral medication I'd be taking for another five years during regular follow up care. While I'd heard mostly about Tamoxifen, Dr. Murphy recommended a newer drug called Arimidex. This was a total estrogen blocker with a little better track record for preventing recurrence. Along with this daily pill I'd need to take Fosamax to strengthen my bones since I would be producing no estrogen for protection against osteoporosis.

Now we turned most all of our attention to the final two weeks of wedding preparations. All my energizing endorphins kicked in while no fewer than 40 friends and relatives contributed their time and talents to making this festive occasion a grand success. Dianne and Julie were at the ready as "gophers" willing to do anything I asked. Three neighbors offered their homes to lodge our out-of-town guests. Katie's beautician cousin, Terri, came from Spokane to style the bridesmaids' hair. Another cousin, David, prepared the music for the reception. The men in Ryan's family became a crew to set up the tent and tables for the outdoor reception. Julie was put in charge of Katie's greyhound, Lexi, who was adorned in a yellow, feather boa collar to match the color scheme of the festivities. Lexi greeted guests at the reception, but was confined to the parking lot during the church ceremony. The outcome was a day of near perfection.

Two weeks after the wedding we were cruising the Rhine from Basel, Switzerland to Amsterdam with Ryan and Katie. Seven months of aggressive cancer treatment was behind me. Though I still had only a fuzzy re-growth of light-colored hair, I felt little discomfort with or without a wig. Once on a breezy afternoon as we viewed the castle-dotted countryside from the upper deck of the ship, Katie and Ryan worried that my wig might blow off in the wind. I think we would all have laughed uproariously if that had happened. Life was too good and too short to worry about appearances and trivialities.

Once docked in Amsterdam, the four of us rented bicycles to ride several days through the Low Countries of Holland and Belgium. Mostly flatlands across these beautiful countries were inviting. We planned to take the train to Bruges, then spend three nights visiting medieval towns as we rode the trails and highways back to Amsterdam. Our departure on this adventure became a most memorable morning as I took a tumble with my bicycle halfway up the escalator in Central Station. I punctured my left knee and broke the little finger on my left hand. To be sure, I had no sense of embarrassment about my lack of hair during the scene where train station personnel gathered around to give first aid and an audience of curious onlookers observed my clumsiness and injuries. Somehow we got to our hotel in the magnificent windmill city of Bruges. Bill biked to a pharmacy where he stumbled with his broken bits of German to purchase some casting materials, bandages and painkillers. It occurred to me how fortunate I was to be traveling with my own orthopedic surgeon! All those precautionary warnings I heard about protecting my compromised left side seemed to no avail. After a drugged-but-restful night's sleep, I was ready to ride again so as not to spoil the honeymoon adventure. Again and again I marveled with gratitude at my good fortune to be so healthy a survivor of breast cancer.

Life continues to happen…thankfully!

As fall, 2004 approached, life settled back into a normal rhythm. Bill traveled with his work several days each week. I focused on completing my memoir before the end of the year. Work at the Habitat store, Tuesdays at Dorle's and church activities resumed at pre-cancer levels. There were still some doctor and dentist appointments, and some follow-up lab tests, but the cancer cloud had dissipated from our lives.

Only in early September, when Dorle's physicians advised her that further treatment was futile, did the gravity of breast cancer hurtle back into my primary consciousness. Dorle, who loved holidays and was well known for decorating her house and yard for every possible festive occasion, decided she wanted the whole town to join her for one last mega celebration. I volunteered to address and send 100 invitations, which drew a huge crowd for a Saturday evening, potluck dinner party. Each room, hallway or distinct area of her house or yard was decorated for a different holiday. Partygoers were invited to select a favorite decoration as they left, a memento from Dorle to symbolize her heartfelt connection with all these friends who had shared these sacred moments of her life with cancer.

In mid-August we'd talked with our friends from Austin about sharing a few days with us after their attendance at a medical meeting in Vancouver, B.C. They had needed to focus primary concern on the declining health of their son whose melanoma was resisting successive courses of difficult treatment, and to support their daughter-in-law and only grandchild as they faced the loss of husband and father. We certainly knew what they were experiencing in awful anticipation of child loss. They would come for the long Labor Day weekend and we would find some marvelous diversions on the beautiful Olympic Peninsula.

A week before they were to depart from Texas, Liz called to discuss final arrangements, and disclosed to me that a mutual close friend in Austin had just been diagnosed with breast cancer. MaryAnna, a widow and single mother, was dealing with the shock over her disease and the demand for her to make critical decisions about her treatment. Liz suggested she call me. MaryAnna worried that she'd be stirring up negative feelings I didn't need to revisit, now that I'd passed through the long journey of surgery, chemo and radiation. Liz told me she'd replied, "MaryAnna, Cheron has gotten through it and she's very upbeat and optimistic. You really should talk with her."

After our phone conversation, MaryAnna and I decided that she should fly to Seattle and join the vacation we'd planned for our foursome. What a poignant time of laughter, love and sharing our deepest emotions, fears, wisdom and common history. The time and conversation we shared served to confirm my growing conviction that all was well and that I should expect to enjoy a few more decades of life.

Shortly thereafter Bill suggested we consider buying a house or condo in Arizona for the winters of our retirement together. And we did. Life began to feel normal again, distancing us each day a little further beyond the fear and foreboding of life with, or death from, cancer. By October we were fully into our former routines of work and play. The manuscript for my book was approaching readiness for submission to peer reviewers, and I began to look for a publisher. Ginger and I were deeply involved in partnering with a very needy family that had been selected to receive a Habitat house. Katie and Ryan had moved to Virginia for the next phase of his Coast Guard assignment, so we took the opportunity to visit them, after which we parlayed the trip into a vacation the four of us shared touring Washington, D.C. We went to a wedding in southern California, which gave us a wonderful opportunity to visit with Ryan's dear parents, whom we had come to cherish as both friends and family. We got back to regular and increasingly vigorous training for the marathon events we'd enjoyed for over a decade in our quest for health and wellness. The Royal Victorian Marathon in British Columbia had become an October tradition, and I observed with satisfaction my ability and excitement about participating in this annual feat, although I chose the shorter 10K walk instead of the 13-mile half marathon competition.

When we met with our insurance agent in late-October for the annual re-evaluation of our health care coverage, I realized that my most aggravating health concern had now become the deterioration of my knees. It had been relegated to the back burner while cancer was in the forefront, but now I reawakened to the pain and limitation imposed by worn-out knees. I almost surprised myself when I determined to go forward with bilateral knee replacement surgery at Thanksgiving time.

Expensive major surgery, pain, and physical therapy...I must be expecting a good many more years of active living! Building a new home in Arizona? Both Bill and I must be feeling confident we'll have plenty of time to enjoy life in the beautiful, sunny Southwest. Friends and others now consulting ME about how to conquer cancer! Despite a year of illness, doubts and challenging decisions, it feels as if I'm back on track and life is truly good. My attitude of gratitude is pervasive again. Thanks be to God, to Bill, to my friends, to the breast cancer sisterhood, to the marvels of medicine and the people who've dedicated their careers to making possible the return to wellness after cancer diagnosis. Yes, life IS good and to be celebrated everyday. Hooray! I'm alive and kickin'!

Printed in the United States
132243LV00001B/5/P